Men in the Lives of Young Children

This book presents an international perspective on the involvement of men in the lives of young children across a range of differing contexts and from a number of disciplinary perspectives. It takes as a starting point the importance of positive male engagement with young children so as to ensure their optimal development. Past research has revealed the complexity of studying these relationships and the barriers that exist in families and society which impede the implementation of positive relationships. This book is developed to use new research and educational thinking in order to explore the lived experiences of both fathers and men in edu-care and also to consider what it is to be a man in the 21st century. As such this work is pertinent, timely and responsive to issues of concern to all those professionals, policy makers and practitioners within education and family services and also to the public in general. The central purpose of the book is to contribute to the debate around key issues connected to the ways in which men can develop secure professional and familial attachments to young children for whom they have a responsibility.

This book was published as a special issue of *Early Child Development and Care*.

Deborah Jones is Reader in Education in the School of Sport and Education at Brunel University in West London. For many years she has co-ordinated teacher education programmes in the initial training of teachers for the early years and pre-secondary phase. She is currently researching the career narratives of men in head teacher roles in early years settings.

Roy Evans is Professor of Education in the School of Sport and Education at Brunel University in West London and was previously Head of the Education Department. His research has focussed on the education of marginalised and special groups of children and those 'at risk' of educational underachievement due to environmental, familial and personal factors.

Men in the Lives of Young Children

An international perspective

Edited by Deborah Jones and Roy Evans

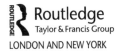
Routledge
Taylor & Francis Group

LONDON AND NEW YORK

First published 2009 by Routledge
2 Park Square, Milton Park, Abingdon, Oxon, OX14 4RN

Simultaneously published in the USA and Canada
by Routledge
711 Third, New York, NY 10017

Routledge is an imprint of the Taylor & Francis Group, an informa business

First issued in paperback 2013

© 2009 Taylor & Francis

Typeset in Plantin by Value Chain, India

British Library Cataloguing in Publication Data
A catalogue record for this book is available from the British Library

ISBN13: 978-0-415-49704-6 (hbk)
ISBN13: 978-0-415-84895-4 (pbk)

CONTENTS

Introduction: Men in caring, parenting and teaching: exploring men's roles with young children

Roy Evans and Deborah Jones
Brunel University, Twickenham, UK

Across the international scene common features consistently occur in relation to men's involvement in the lives of young children. There have been repeated government initiatives to attract more men into educare contexts (Mills et al., 2004) while developing father's interest in young children have also been on the agenda. However such enterprises have not always been straightforward. At a transnational level difficulties have arisen with regard to both recruitment and retention of males in early childhood contexts and 'father's programmes' have had a chequered history. Such initiatives have taken place against a background of many conflicting discourses. For example, it is perceived that the teaching profession is 'in crisis' due to the lack of male teachers. The feminisation of primary teaching is seen to be detrimental—to male pupils in particular (Bleach, 1998; Johannesson, 2004). This view has been promulgated by media, teaching unions and governments alike. Equally, within the public discourse there are oppositional strands. Males in educare must cope with discourses of both risk and adulation. On the one hand, they are hailed as important male role models in a society where absentee fathers are prevalent. On the other, they are subject to suspicion manifested both in homophobia or accusations of abuse. They are perceived variously as super-heroes or demons, the latter being by far the strongest discourse (Jones, 2007). All men who enter and stay in such professions have to deal with suspicion it appears (Martino & Berrill, 2003) and may at certain points be perceived as 'high risk' (McWilliam & Jones, 2005).The effect is to effectively keep the numbers of men in educare contexts down.

Within postmodern society the cultural construction of masculinity together with patriarchal assumptions about gendered identities have been challenged. There has been a so-called 'crisis in masculinity', where the concept of a single fixed unified masculinity is difficult to justify. Rather, for men, multiple identities/masculinities are on offer from which they may choose. The concepts of hybridised, bricolage masculinity are presented whereby men may 'channel hop' across versions of the masculine according to need (Beynon, 2002). However, besides opening up certain freedoms for men, tensions also result from the multiplicity of identities presented.

For example, although it may be maintained that men are capable of caring for young children (King, 2005) close involvement may be perceived as the prerogative of women, who are widely held as being 'better for the job' and dominate the caring professions. Linked to this and prevalent within the public discourse is the denigration of involvement with young children as 'women' work', while dominant forms of male heterosexuality are characterised by the need to avoid closeness in relationships and to fear emotions (Kimmel, 1994; Connell, 2005) neither of which are called for in early childhood settings. Such disparate discourses impact and present difficulties for men in contemporary society.

This book presents an international perspective on the involvement of men in the lives of young children across a range of differing contexts. It explores the lived experiences of both fathers and men in educare and in addition considers what it is to be a man in the twenty-first century. As such this collection is pertinent, timely and responds to issues which are of concern to those within educare, to those within families and also to the public in general.

In the initial chapter, Alice Honig provides a comprehensive review of research on fathering together with research on men employed in work with young children. Both centres and elementary schools as places of work are considered. Throughout, Honig emphasises the importance of positive male engagement with young children for their optimal development. She notes however, that research reveals the complexity of studying these relationships and that barriers in families and society exist which impede the implementation of positive interactions. Within this chapter, suggestions are given for increasing positive male participation in the home and in educational settings.

Deborah Jones presents research undertaken with male headteachers in early years schools within the UK and explores several influencial discourses in relation to male headteachers' identities. The chapter discusses the ways in which different identities are constructed for headteachers by parents, governors and wider society and also how a variety of discourses impact on men's' professional lives. Jones examines themes inherent in headteachers' discourses as they reflect upon their roles and experiences within the school context and consider the practice of identity construction. She notes that tensions are increased as a result of multiple, frequently conflicting identities for example the pressure to present both distant and caring personae. The chapter concludes by acknowledging that the role of headship functions to protect men from the denigration to which other male teachers are sometimes subjected. However, the role may operate to distance them from the closer relationships which they frequently desire. As such being a male headteacher is characterised by complexity.

Michel Vandenbroeck and Jan Peeters's paper on gender and professionalism draws attention to gender segregation in the caring professions. They note that research and experiments so far show that it may take decades of multiple actions to overcome the gender divide in the caring workforce. However, research that includes the voices of men in child care is rather recent, scarce and involves only very small samples of male carers. Therefore, they suggest, little is known about the students' perspectives on how the gendered culture of the profession is transmitted through overt or covert curricula and how this may affect them. By means of three studies the authors begin to unveil how future male carers are affected by both overt and covert gendered curricula. A first study interviewed 30 students in initial training, while a second study involved 16 men in adult education for caring professions. A third study examined 1635 pages of textbooks. Together the studies show how both overt and covert curricula affect younger students more than their adult colleagues and how persistent, long-term strategies are needed to attract both men and women into the care workforce.

Mary Thornton and Patricia Bricheno provide a particular focus on men in teaching. They note that the number of males in teaching has always been small, particularly in early childhood. Nevertheless those that do enter the profession usually do so for the same reasons as women, namely enjoyment of working with children, wanting to teach and wanting to make a difference to children's lives. However, in two separate studies Thornton and Bricheno (2006) have shown that on beginning teacher training in 1998, and at the point of leaving the profession in 2005, men and women tend to emphasise different concerns. This chapter explores those differences and seeks possible explanations for how men's views of teaching might be changing over time.

Sarah-Eve Farquhar explores New Zealand men's participation in early years work and notes that the history of kiwi men's participation in paid early child care and teaching work has not been documented to date. Farquhar argues that what can be learned from the New Zealand experience may be helpful internationally in the movement towards greater male representation in early years work. Therefore, this paper provides a brief recent history, highlighting issues that may be specific to New Zealand's cultural and political context as well as those likely to be generic to men's experiences within any western country.

A review of the literature on father involvement in early childhood programmes is presented by Glen Palm and Jay Fagan. They acknowledge that father involvement in early childhood programmes has increased rapidly during the past 10–15 years. This chapter reviews their understanding of the current state of father involvement in early childhood programmes and in so doing, employs two theoretical frameworks: ecological perspective and situated fathering. Palm and Fagan draw from the research and practice literature to understand the current levels of father involvement in early education programmes, the factors that support this type of father involvement, the barriers to father involvement and strategies for increasing father involvement in early childhood programmes.

The paper by Carol Potter and John Carpenter presents a case study from the UK, of one Sure Start programme's significant success in engaging large numbers of fathers with its services. The paper details both the levels of male involvement in the programme over time and the strategies found to be effective in involving men. Numbers of fathers using programme services rose to over 100 in 2005, with the total number of male attendances exceeding 1000 in that same year. The successful engagement of fathers in this programme's activities was found to be as a result of a combination of both strategic and day to day approaches. Effective strategic approaches were close partnership working with an expert local voluntary agency, the use of a gender differentiated approach and in-going commitment to the work at programme management level. Factors related to success at a day-to-day level included the high level of skill and persistence demonstrated by a dedicated father worker and the implicit use of a social marketing approach. Throughout, Potter and Carpenter discuss findings in the context of current national policy contexts relating to father engagement.

Flora Macleod contributes an important perspective on why fathers are not attracted to family learning groups. She notes that accounts of fathers' reluctance to engage with locally based family learning groups rarely acknowledge the relationship between learning and identity. This tends not to be the case in parallel accounts of women's reluctance to become involved in groups or networks where the mainstream clientele is male. Drawing on the case study of a national initiative aimed at developing family literacy in local communities throughout the UK, Macleod argues that decisions to join or not to join these groups is primarily social and cultural rather than individual. This means that the attendance of fathers at family learning events needs to be understood in context. It also means addressing the complexities underpinning their reasons for not attending from a lifelong perspective. When this approach is taken the implications for policy and practice become clearer. What works for some will not work for others. Rather than relying on a standard provision for all, what is needed suggests Macleod, is a range of high quality dedicated provision that caters for different requirements, specifically in this case, the differing needs and preferences of mothers and fathers.

Lisa Newland, Diana Coyl and Harry Freeman take predicting preschoolers attachment security as their focus. Associations between preschoolers' attachment security, fathers' involvement (i.e. parenting behaviours and consistency) and father-ing context (i.e. fathers' internal working models and use of social support) were examined in a subsample of 102 fathers, taken from a larger sample of 235 culturally diverse US families. The authors' predicted that fathers' involvement would mediate associations between children's attachment security and less proximal fathering context. Fathers completed questionnaires regarding their parenting behaviours, internal working models of adult relationships, their use of social support and an attachment Q-List to assess their preschoolers' attachment security. Fathers' involve-ment mediated the relationship between fathering context and children's attachment security. Newland et al. discuss the ways in which their findings support an ecological view of children's attachment security within a multilayered system.

The paper by Harry Freeman, Lisa Newland and Diana Coyl explores fathers' beliefs as a mediator between contextual barriers and father involvement. They exam-ine fathers' beliefs as mediators between multiple risk factors and involvement prac-tices with children age from 0 to 5 enrolled in Head Start or Early Head Start. As part of their research, a diverse sample of 101 fathers, living in rural midwestern commu-nities of the USA completed questionnaires assessing *mediators* (i.e. parenting effi-cacy, role beliefs and responsibility to an intervention programme), *barriers* (e.g. lack of time, energy, work constraints) and *father involvement* (i.e. physical play, didactic engagement, caregiving, socialisation, involvement in the programme and accessibility). In each of the regression models, father efficacy and beliefs reduced the influence of barriers and were significant unique predictors of father involvement. Findings suggest that fathers' beliefs are more proximal to parenting practices than is family context. Freeman et al. explore the implications of their research for early intervention programmes specifically serving children in at-risk families.

Bernard Spodek and Olivia Saracho's chapter discusses studies that provide the historical and contemporary patterns of father involvement in the USA. In this way researchers are provided with an understanding of contemporary fatherhood. Spodek and Saracho describe the historical patterns and research on father involvement that created methodological and conceptual challenges in conducting studies that characterise fathers. A number of frequent measurement approaches, challenges and limitations that are found in such studies are presented and discussed. The chapter concludes with recommendations for future research and practical applications that can guide researchers to improve their studies on fathers and to better understand the complexity of fatherhood.

Olivia Saracho takes as her focus fathers and young children's literacy experiences. A family literacy programme was investigated to document the literacy experiences of 25 fathers and their five-year-old children. Using a case study methodology, she examined the effects of a literacy intervention that was designed to assist fathers to promote their children's acquisition of literacy. The results indicated that the fathers who learn literacy strategies and related activities can contribute to their children's literacy development. Fathers in the literacy intervention programme received the same literacy instruction, but they modified the instruction not only to their own personal style, but also to the literacy strategies, interactions, materials and activities that they learned. The trends and innovations in the literacy programme related to the teaching–learning process and their collaboration. Saracho emphasises that both trends and innovations indicated that the fathers could make important contributions to their children's literacy development.

In the final chapter, John Barker considers men and motors and the ways in which fathers are involved in children's travel. He notes that while there is a growing body of literature considering the different settings in which young children spend their time, less explored is how children travel to and from the different everyday spaces of childhood. Although research on gendered carescapes has identified the central role of mothers in caring for and escorting children, as well as the changing role of fathers, little attention has been paid to the role of and expectations of fathers in relation to undertaking these escorting tasks. Drawing upon research conducted in the UK with young children and their families, Barker contributes to existing debates by exploring the role of fathers in escorting children to a variety of settings, considering how fathers may have diverse experiences of escorting. He also explores how cars play a particularly important role for fathers' escort of children, and how fathers' involvement may create particular masculine styles of caring which are distinctive from those children experience with mothers.

References

Beynon, J. (2002) *Masculinities and culture* (Buckingham, Open University Press).

Bleach, K. (Ed.) (1998) *Raising boys' achievement in school* (Stoke-on-Trent, Trentham).

Connell, R. W. (2005) *Masculinities* (Berkeley, CA, University of California Press).

Johannesson, I. A. (2004) To teach boys and girls: a pro-feminist perspective on the boy's debate in Iceland, *Educational Review*, 56(1), 33–41.

Jones, D. (2007) Millennium man: constructing identities of male teachers in early years contexts, *Educational Review*, 59(2), 179–194.

Kimmel, M. S. (1994) Masculinity as homophobia: fear, shame, and silence in the construction of gender identity, in: H. Brod & M. Kaufman (Eds) *Theorizing Masculinities* (Thousand Oaks, CA, Sage), 119–141.

King, J. R. (2005) *Uncommon caring: learning from men who teach young children* (Columbia University, New York/London, Teachers College Press).

Martino, W. & Berrill, D. (2003) Boys, schooling and masculinities: interrogating the 'right' way to educate boys, *Education Review*, 55(2), 99–117.

Mills, M., Martino, W. & Lingard, B. (2004) Attracting, recruiting and retaining male teachers: policy issues in the male teacher debate, *British Journal of Sociology of Education*, 25(3), 355–369.

McWilliam, E. & Jones, A. (2005) An unprotected species? On teachers as risky subjects, *British Educational Research Journal*, 31(1), 109–120.

Thornton, M. & Bricheno, P. (2006) *Missing men in education* (Stoke-on-Trent, Trentham).

Supporting men as fathers, caregivers, and educators

Alice Sterling Honig

College of Human Ecology, Syracuse University, New York, USA

For decades, research on men's influence on children focused on concerns for worrisome educational and socio-emotional effects of father absence, particularly in families living in poverty (Biller, 1970). Fatherless children are five times more likely to live in poverty than children living with both parents. 'Violent criminals are overwhelmingly males who grew up without fathers—60% of America's rapists, 72% of adolescent murderers, and 70% of long-term prison inmates' (Bradley, 1998, p. D3). Children in father-absent families are reported to have lower educational achievements, more aggression, and less self-regulation.

In earlier centuries:

> Fathers were viewed as all-powerful patriarchs who wielded enormous power over their families. Fathers were primarily responsible for ensuring that their children grew up with an appropriate sense of values, acquired primarily from a study of the Bible ... Around the time of industrialization, however, primary focus shifted from moral leadership to breadwinning and economic support of the family. Then, perhaps as a result of the Great

Depression, which revealed many men as poor providers, social scientists came to portray fathers as sex-role models .... In contrast to earlier conceptualizations of fathers' roles, researchers, theorists, and practitioners ... recognize that fathers play a number of significant roles—companions, care provider's spouses, protectors, models, moral guides, teachers, breadwinners—whose relative importance varies across historical epochs and subcultural groups. (Lamb & Tamis-LeMonda, 2004, pp. 3–4)

Textbooks on child development until recently have not given much space to father–child relationships over time and as a function of often complex modern family relationships and childcare settings. One recent popular text, for example, devotes just a couple of pages—only to father involvement in childbirth, adjustment following the birth of a baby, and the option of paternity leave!

Yet recent decades have seen an explosive growth and interest in many nations in father/child research (Tamis-LeMonda & Cabrera, 2002). Studies have delved more deeply and also more broadly into the whole gamut of male interactions with infants and children across many societies, and focused on paternal influences in relation to a wide range of outcomes, including peer relationships and even children's ability when grown to adulthood to bond affectionately with their own infants (Lamb, 2004).

Researchers into men's impact on children's lives have a difficult job! Men are now interacting with children not only as biological parents in the home, but also as divorced dads living apart from their children's residence. Men are interacting with children in a variety of other relationships—as stepfathers, grandfathers, foster fathers, and partners with women who already have children. Some fathers live with biological *and* with stepchildren. Some men work with children in educational institutions, such as childcare and elementary grades. Some work in special settings for children with disabilities. Some fathers are violent toward their children and also live in violent neighborhoods, while others try to shield their children from the violence in their environment and on the television (Fitzgerald *et al.*, 2006).

Researchers have been particularly eager to emphasize the need to focus on *positive* paternal involvement (Palkovitz, 2002). But how shall positive paternal involvement be defined? Pleck (1997) has urged that father involvement be conceptualised with emphasis on positive paternal involvement, defined as 'high engagement, accessibility and responsibility ... not just "going through the motions" of fatherhood'(p. 102). Study of men's involvement with their children should emphasise their 'positive, wide-ranging, and active participation in their children's lives' (Marsiglio *et al.*, 2000, p. 276).

McKeown *et al.* (1998) explain that authoritative fathering 'which involves providing consistent values and boundaries and relating to the child with warmth and confidence, is beneficial to the child, but "authoritarian" fathering, which involves excessive discipline, control, and aloofness from the child, is not' (p. 87).

Fathers, who remembered that their own fathers had been high in expressing anger and low in expressing love, themselves had children who were rated as more aggressive and hyperactive in kindergarten (Cowan *et al.*, 1996).

Case studies and qualitative research findings often are helpful in furthering understanding of *positive paternal involvement*. As Piburn (2006) has noted 'Perhaps the clearest evidence of global change lies less in evolving workforce statistics, and more in the numbers of men in public with infants strapped to their chests, pushing strollers on the street, and at the diaper changing tables inside men's restrooms at restaurants, malls, and airports'(p. 18).

One of the winning entries written for a Father's Day contest in which wives nominated the 'Best Dad Ever' provides a poignant example of how rich case studies can be for understanding fathering behaviors:

> In our world, a normal dad golfs, watches sports, goes four-wheeling with buddies, and works late. My husband, Michael, does none of these things. He says our children are his life. He is truly an angel among dads. I have never seen a father who is as gentle as he is. He has never raised his voice or his hand to them. His childhood was filled with hitting, yelling, and throwing, and he is determined that his children never know violence. I suffer from depression, severe sometimes; my husband just picks up the slack—without complaining. He sleeps in our baby's room and takes care of her all night so I can sleep. Then he goes to work early so he can come home early and help me with our kids. His work is stressful. He is a religious educator for high school students; some of whom are special needs kids. He never brings his work home or complains. Our children have emulated his unfailing optimism and hardworking nature. His favorite pastime truly is playing with the kids and reading to them. All you have to do is look at our children to know what kind of father he is. They are the most respectful and helpful children I have even known. For these and many other reasons, I believe he is the best dad in the world. (Phelps, 2008, p. 86)

Amount of time spent often was used as a measure of father involvement. But this may not be a good predictive measure for positive child outcomes. Indeed, researchers no longer focus just on amount of time a father is available to a child!

> Simply being there is not enough; being available and involved is what really counts .... kids whose fathers are cold and authoritarian, derogatory and intrusive have the hardest time with grades and social relationships. They are even worse off than kids who live in homes with no father at all. Kids with non-supportive dads and dads who humiliate them were the ones .... most likely to be headed for trouble. They were the ones who displayed aggressive behavior toward their friends, they were the ones who had trouble in school, and they were the ones with problems often linked to delinquency and youth violence. (Parke & Brott, 1999, pp. 9–10)

Further variables to consider in studying fathering

Subtle variables need to be considered in inquiring into paternal styles and child outcomes.

Age when paternity begins

Children of *teen fathers* may be at greater risk not only for psychological outcomes but for physical risks, such as 'shaken baby syndrome,' in comparison with infants born to mature parents. Some fathers in new marriages have started second families at a much later age. Paternal late childrearing may be very different from earlier patterns. There are risks and benefits for late childrearing. Paternal age over 40 is associated medically with higher risk of fathering children with rare mutations and more complex disorders, such as autism or schizophrenia (Saey, 2008). Paternal age may have a vital influence on patterns of interactions for a number of reasons, including more paternal *reflectiveness* about having played a distant or negligible role as a parent with children from a first marriage and a resolution to be a more engaged and sensitive father in the new family.

Father interactions when alone with child or with mother present

In a Swedish study, fathers were more likely to display affectionate behavior and engage in more play with their 8–12-month-old infants when alone with their babies and mothers were not present (Hwang, 1986). Studies of fathers need to take note of such possible differences when observing the quality of paternal interactions.

Intergenerational changes in fathering

The Internet and television have increased the possibility for dissemination of new ideas and versions of family life across the world. Despite the slowness with which particular cultural taboos or mores change in some cultures, increased global access to the Web could enhance the possibility of more intergenerational changes in paternal parenting styles in some societies.

Electronic information sharing across the globe supports the importance of conducting ongoing *longitudinal* research. For example, in traditional Korean culture, fathers were far more involved with sons than with daughters. Parental roles reflected the Confucian classic rule 'a stern male and a nurturant female' (Yi, 1993, p. 19). Yi explains that the household was divided into two sectors, and men and women were rigidly separated. The husband was referred to as *bagatyangban,* the person who is exterior, and the wife was referred to as *anae,* the person who is interior. After age 5, boys moved to the men's quarters, and their mothers taught girls domestic responsibilities. No contact or communication was permitted between males and females, even for seven-year-old children. Modern Korean culture has shifted from this gender-rigid patterning of parenting roles and responsibilities. In intergenerational interviews with Korean male family adults, regarding how they handle developmentally normative behaviors and how they discipline young children, fathers reported more flexible and empathic involvement with both male and female children compared with responses of their own fathers (the children's grandfathers) about how they had interacted with their preschool children (Jung & Honig, 2001).

Cross-cultural researches are very important in adding to knowledge of men's interactions with children. Father involvement with infants and young children varies markedly across culture groups. Cross-cultural data on paternal investment indicates that 'father involvement is lowest in African cultures, while it is highest in Southeast Asian and Pacific Island Cultures' (Hewlitt, 2004, p. 187).

One vivid example of the importance of gathering cross-cultural data is that rough and tumble play was considered important as a fathering technique in recent research in the USA. But inquiry into father interactions with very young children in other cultures has found that this is not a way that fathers interact with their young children at all in some societies. Aka hunter-gatherers in the African Republic are gentle, highly engaged, and physically nurturing with their children. Hewlitt (2004) reports that:

> ... because Aka fathers knew their infants so well, they did not have to use vigorous play to initiate communication or interactions ... [and they] show their love in other ways ... Aka fathers knew how to read and understand their infants' verbal and nonverbal communication. (p. 189)

Social class

Not only culture, but also *social class* is an important variable in studying men's patterns of interaction with infants and young children. Replies from African-American fathers from different social classes as to how they responded to child requests and to developmentally normative or unapproved behaviors of their preschoolers, revealed that middle class African-American fathers' patterns of responses with both male and female preschoolers were quite similar to those of White middle class respondents, but differed in some domains from responses provided by low-education African-American fathers who were living in poverty (Honig & Mayne, 1982).

Education as a powerful contributor to positive parenting

Findings from the sixth National Survey of Family Growth in the USA reported that education was a key factor in fatherhood and the main predictor of a father's positive involvement with his children. Fathers who had been to college, in comparison with fathers who had a high school diploma or less, were more likely to eat meals with or feed children under five every day (78.6% vs. 70.3%). They were more likely to bathe, diaper, and dress small children (66.4% vs. 43.6%). They were more likely to play with children every day (87.1% vs. 75.8%). Of particular importance for children's readiness for school, highly educated fathers were more likely to read to children each day (32% vs. 9.5%) (www.cdc.gov/nchs/dataa/series/sr_23/sr_026.pdf).

Effects of father's attachment history in his family of origin

Attachment of infants to mothers has been intensively studied for over half a century since Bowlby's pioneer observations in England and Ainsworth's establishment in Baltimore of the Strange Situation as the predominant technique for assessing infant attachment to a caregiver. 'Secure attachment' is defined as a strong emotional bond between a baby or young child and a nurturing, tuned-in caregiver. Secure attachment develops through the infant's experiences and interactions during the first year with key adult caregivers. Attachment representations, whether secure or insecure, become internalized working models. They are 'templates that serve as guides for interpreting emotions, perceptions, and behaviors in all future relationships' (Honig, 2002, p. 4).

Intergenerational transmission of security of attachment has been confirmed in longitudinal researches in several societies. The impact of the quality of emotional relationships with parents that a father has had in his own family of origin *does* impact on the quality of attachment that develops between his baby and himself. Infants at one year tend to have less secure relationships with fathers who report poor emotional relations in childhood with their own parents (Steele *et al.*, 1996). The dads were interviewed *prior* to the birth of the baby. Thus, a positive advance in our knowledge of men's involvement with the children they care for is that attachment research now actively focuses on the *attachment of infants to fathers* as well as to mothers.

Fathers who perceive their own importance in their infants' development, who show delight in, as well as sensitivity to the needs of their babies at three months, and who consider it very important to spend time with their babies are more likely to have one-year-olds who are securely attached to them (Cox *et al.*, 1992).

Gender unease between men and women

Some of the perplexity about how to involve more fathers in intimate nurturing interactions with their children or how to increase the recruitment of males into nursery work rests on discomforts that each gender has with what are perceived as the work 'domains' of the other. Caring for infants and young children has been traditionally perceived as 'women's work'—an idea still deeply regarded as a truism in many culture groups in the world.

This gender discomfort is vividly expressed by Ian, a trained male nursery teacher in Great Britain, as he muses about how working class fathers actually feel and perceive his nursery classroom:

> When they come in and it's all nice pink pastel colours and flowers and women are walking around everywhere, middle class women, the children, all 26 children are screaming, and they're all painting and paint brushes everywhere ... I got to think that this guy has worked 20 years in shipyard, he's just become unemployed. I know his child's on free dinners. What is in it for him at the center? In that situation there is nothing ... he's gonna feel threatened you know. There's nothing for him when he does come. He's not gonna feel comfortable. So I can see why people do sport and digging and school trips. It's a great way for blokes to get involved and to feel comfortable. But we've also got to work on building up the relationship with the parents and the fathers so that you can make that next step and get involved with actual education, the care of the child, and develop that partnership thing. (Warin, 2006, p. 527)

Ian developed a variety of musical strategies to involve fathers—including a Father's Band, and an all-male singing group. He revealed that in the singing group, dads could comment about some of the *pleasures of fathering*, which they would not be able to risk talking about at other male social settings, such as watching football or at the work place. Ian explained:

> How often do men get a chance to go somewhere in a group and say 'my children are quite wonderful actually' and *say* that to someone, 'cause you don't do it at the pub ... When else do you get a chance to say actually 'I'm dead chuffed my son's gone to the toilet for the first time by himself? (Warin, 2006, p. 528)

Working parents

Dual- and single-earner families present special challenges in devising strategies for studying and encouraging paternal involvement with children. Work choices by parents affect child–father intimate relationships. A higher proportion of insecure attachments between sons and fathers (but not daughters) has been reported in dual-earner, compared with single-earner families (Chase-Lansdale & Owen, 1987; Belsky & Rovine, 1988).

Grych and Clark (1999) note that although greater father participation in caregiving is associated with enhanced cognitive and social development in children, participation that is *required*, as in dual-career families, may not have as sanguine results. They speculate that in dual-earner households, some fathers do not feel they have much control over the obligation to be responsible for more daily childcare tasks before they feel ready or able to do so. Thus, they experience greater stress and frustration that leads to less sensitive or responsive parenting. Of interest in this study is that at 12 months, fathers exhibited significantly more positive effect and behaviors with their female infants than with sons. Fathers with non-employed wives showed higher levels of involvement with greater expressed positive affect, sensitivity, and responsiveness compared with fathers whose wives worked more than 25 hours per week. When mothers were not employed or employed part time, then fathers also expressed higher levels of marital satisfaction when the babies were four months old and later, at one year of age. *Marital satisfaction* is another variable that must be assessed when studying differential paternal interactions with young children.

Fathers' gender role ideology

In a study of preschoolers' parents' views on male role norms and parental roles, the more time that fathers spent as the child's primary caregiver, the more likely were the fathers to report more liberal views of the father's role. 'Active participation in childcare appears to reinforce fathers' belief that they are as well-suited and as important for childcare as their wives' (Bonney *et al.*, 1999, p. 411). Further, men performed more childcare tasks among couples where there was *high marital satisfaction*. One pathway toward increasing father involvement might lie in *offering counseling to families to resolve marital issues* where high intensity conflicts serve as a major deterrent to fathers' positive engagement with and care for their young children.

Effects of parental job loss

Financial uncertainties attendant upon job loss, as well as increased paternal worries, provoke stresses and strains in father–child relationships. During the Great Depression in the USA, relations between fathers and children were affected by the frustrations and discouragements of fathers who had previously been breadwinners for the family (Elder, 1974). Youths (children born in 1920–21) suffered negative education, achievement, and health effects into adulthood. In this sample from working-class families, female children who were physically attractive seemed buffered from paternal negative interactions.

Perceived gender differences in power

'Power is the ability to influence others, to be listened to, to get your way rather than having to do what others want' (Tannen, 2001, p. 317). Men have historically been perceived as more powerful than women.

Head Start providers, interviewed in the Beach Center study, frequently raised the issue of differential power relationships between men and women (Turbiville *et al.*, 2000). Based on their own personal experiences of domestic violence, some of the women care providers felt anger over the physical presence of fathers, despite training programs to increase gender sensitivity. When interviewed for this study, the fathers themselves expressed eager interest in employment training opportunities or classroom work with the children when compared with fathers in other studies.

Because of power differentials, some theoreticians (Kelly, 1998) see men's more extensive engagement in childcare as problematic and even of possible concern unless:

> That engagement is set in a wider context of men's anti-oppressive practice. This involves men challenging dominant relations of power in the family, welfare services, and society more generally. If such a broader practice is not implemented, then men's greater engagement in childcare by itself may simply result in replication of oppressive power relations in one form or another: annexation or colonization of initiatives development by/for women; diversion of resources away from other initiatives promoting the well-being of women and/ or children; perhaps even abuse of women and/or children (p. 174).

Concerns such as these must be addressed as well as giving due attention to the concerns of male workers who express feeling 'marginalized' working in a world of mostly female care providers.

What further data are needed to promote paternal involvement?

Disentangling specific paternal or male influences on child development outcomes requires in-depth and specific information both quantitative *and* qualitative. Interviewing males about the number of hours they spend in different childcare domains, such as physical childcare (bathing, diapering, or feeding), play, discipline, or administrative tasks with children (arranging for dentist visits or play dates) may not capture the *quality* of the child's relationship with the parent.

One preschooler told me that when her mommy is at work and her daddy takes care of her, he sits in the living room and watches TV and locks her in the bedroom and does not seem to hear her even when she calls out that she needs to go to the toilet! Yet that time might be counted as 'number of father hours spent with child without mother present.' Another child reported happily that her daddy (Mom's new boyfriend) pushes her on the swing in a local park. Research that only focuses on the relationship and activities of biological dads with children would not capture the relationship (short-lived as it turned out to be) of this preschooler with a positive non-biologically related male adult role model.

Father absence

Absence of the biological father in the home does not always mean that a child has no father figure. Thus, research will need to inquire about the role of a grandpa, an uncle, or other long-term male role models in the child's life. It is of note that father-less families continue to be the focus for researchers, since desertion, divorce, and the choice for single parenthood result in children living without male role models in many families (Furstenberg *et al.*, 1987). Researchers studying fatherless children over the past decades have reported worrisome effects, such as violence in male children, worsening school behaviors, difficulties with peers, and poor life choices (Federal Interagency Forum on Child and Family Statistics, 1998). Effects of father loss through desertion have been noted to be more deleterious than loss of father due to death (Maier & Lachman, 2000). A child experiencing parental divorce may have lived through extreme hostility and fighting *prior* to the parents' separation. Lamb (2002) has cogently pointed out that father absence may affect children for a *multitude* of reasons. Without a father in the home, a child may not only lack a male model or disciplinarian, but also be living in economically poorer circumstances, with a stressed mother who needs to work more outside the home and thus cannot provide adequate guidance and supervision. The mother may be preoccupied with bitterness and grief and be unable to provide the nurturing comfort the child needs to cope with the rupture in family relationships.

Head Start, the most widely known federal program for families of preschool children living in poverty in the USA, mandates parent involvement. Yet less than half of Head Start children live with both mother and father. Data from Head Start confirm that when fathers were indeed more involved, *whether they lived in the home or not*, then the children exhibited more positive behaviors, had fewer behavior problems, less aggression and less hyperactivity (Administration for Children and Families, 2006, p. 9).

Techniques differ for data collection on father involvement

Interviews are an excellent technique for gathering data on parent–child relationships. Yet, fathering researches often use *mothers as informants* if the father is unavailable for direct requests for interviews. A mother, who has intense resentment for the biological father for abandoning the family, sometimes even prior to the baby's birth, may give a distorted picture of the biological father's attempts to see or interact with the child.

Distortion of maternal information provided may not be related to social class at all. In a personal case, as a licensed psychologist, I testified in court in favor of equal time with the children for a dad whom I had observed in my office as sensitive, gentle and responsively attuned in interactions with his young children. Yet the mother wanted the court to forbid the father from seeing the children for at least six years. As a successful professional herself, she told me that she perceived the father as a 'weak-ling' and wanted him deprived of all parental visitation rights. Using only maternal reports sometimes may not provide as reliable information on fathers' positive emotional investment and skills with his young children.

Mothers, however, may well be critical in assisting researchers to access fathers for interviews and observations. The Early Head Start (EHS) Father Studies relied heavily on mothers for enlisting resident and non-resident biological and non-biolog-ical fathers into their national study of low-income fathers. With the inauguration of EHS, serving children younger than three years in the USA, these studies were launched to examine fathering behaviors in the low-income families whose infants and toddlers were being served in EHS programs across the USA. These studies began in 1997 and were designed to complement the EHS Research and Evaluation Project, which involved random assignment of 30,001 families receiving EHS services. Results were reported in a series of articles published in the journal *Parenting: Science and Practice*, April–September, 2006. In one of the studies, low-income fathers were asked:

> (1) 'What does being a 'good father' mean to you?' (2) 'How has becoming a father impacted your life?' (3) 'Talk about your experiences with your own father.' (4) 'What kinds of help or support do you get to do your job as a father?' (5) 'What gets in the way of being a father?' (6) 'What are you proudest of about your child?' (Summers *et al.*, 2006, p. 148)

Fathers saw themselves as a source of stability (being there for the children), provid-ing support, as a mentor and teacher, guiding, shaping values, teaching children, and serving as a good example of someone to look up to. It should be emphasised that these fathers were accessed through the mothers and therefore had either neutral or positive relationships with the mothers. Many of these men described their own fathers as having been emotionally distant, too busy, or unable to express feelings.

The EHS fathers' positive responses remind us that counselors working with dads, who never experienced good relationships with fathers in their own families of origin, can help their male clients to heal from years of yearning by supporting them in becoming the kind of father to their own little ones that they themselves wished they had had in early childhood.

Another research project in this EHS publication teased out negative and positive clusters of parent behaviors. Cluster analysis was carried out on videotaped father–infant interactions coded at 24 and 36 months (Ryan *et al.*, 2006). Fathers who exhibited behaviors in the negative cluster were more intrusive than they were stimu-lating or sensitive. Toddlers with highly supportive parents had higher Bayley Mental Development Index (MDI) scores than children in the non-supportive cluster groups. By 36 months, children of highly supportive fathers scored significantly higher by 10.3 points on the MDI compared with children of high-negative fathers. The researchers concluded that children of two supportive (rather than detached, negative, or intrusive) parents scored higher than children with only one. Positive father behaviors, not only those of mothers, contributed toward 36-month higher child cognitive outcomes.

Of interest among the findings of the researchers for the National Survey of EHS Fathers is the indication that *two distinct styles of father involvement* appear to be emerging. Programs seem either to emphasize *parenting* or they emphasize men's *personal development* with themes based on provision of training, education, literacy, support, and sports (Raikes & Bellotti, 2006, p. 240). It will certainly be of interest to see whether one or another of these program styles results in more positive outcomes for children. Despite national funding and vigorous efforts, the studies found 'that it is not easy to productively engage fathers; and social programs aimed at supporting families may need to consider additional strategies to make programs more attractive to and supportive of fathers' (Boller *et al.*, 2006, p. 137).

Other in-depth interview studies with low-income African-American fathers have provided richly nuanced data (Nelson *et al.*, 2002). Fathers mentioned that the mothers of their children refused to let them have access to the children, often citing drug dealing, incarceration history, alcoholism, and failure to provide funds for needed items, such as crib or diapers. Many of these fathers did credit their children with motivating them to move from criminal to more mainstream employment and 'to leave their fast and dangerous street lives for more conventional ones' (Nelson *et al.*, 2002, p. 551). The researchers conclude:

> In short, children did a lot for fathers. However, fathers sometimes did very little for their children in return, particularly as these children aged. Oftentimes, fathers described bleak scenarios in which they were barred from fulfilling the fathering role because of their economic marginality and personal problems (drug addiction, for example). Fathers sometimes said that when they could not contribute, they felt too guilty to have ongoing contact with their children. (p. 551)

Differences in maternal and paternal perceptions of father roles and contributions

Researchers need to take into account the possibility that mothers may perceive paternal involvement quite differently from fathers and either actively support or try to prevent it. Research on *differences* in maternal and paternal perceptions are of interest, since increased disparity of perceptions about degree of spousal involvement in childcare activities can lead to more marital friction and thus subsequently to more child distress. Honig and Matsushita (in preparation) found that mothers reported lower satisfaction with paternal degree of involvement in comparison with fathers' satisfaction with mothers' involvement in childcare activities, in varied domains such as play, physical caregiving, administrative planning for child's appointments, reading/teaching and emotional/social interactions.

Observations in the home

In-home observation is a costly and time-consuming method to gather data on paternal involvement. In addition, what has been labeled with moms as the 'girdle on' effect may prevent the investigator from gaining a valid in-home picture of family dynamics. A parent may be on best behavior when a 'stranger' enters the home. One mom in her counseling session confided that her husband was easily angered and used many curse words while disciplining the children. The Home Visitor to this family, however, had not heard the father using strings of angry curse words or seen him get physically violent with his son in her presence. She was puzzled about the mother's complaint that the child had a 'foul mouth' at home. Yet the school principal was complaining to the mother about the child's inappropriate use of curse words and impulsive physical attack on a peer who had teased him out on the playground. The father had been brought up to be strictly obedient to his parents. He wanted the same behaviors from his own children. He considered therapeutically positive suggestions such as using 'I statements' instead of 'You accusatory statements' as just 'psychobabble.' He informed the Home Visitor that it was too hard for him to change; he just wanted the *child* to shape up! Long-term building of trust between outreach workers with families and increased training and skill building for work with parents are important considerations. A Home Visitor needs a large repertoire of techniques to work with parents as well as with a child, if the goal is to promote positive child behavior changes over time (Honig, 1979, 1996).

Since many paternal interactions occur when the father comes home from work, *observational* data on male interactions may be hard to come by. One ingenious researcher confirmed how strong a linguistic influence a loving father can have (and how powerful babies are as language learners) by putting a microphone for a week in the crib of a baby whose papa spoke Spanish with him for a while each day on returning home from work. This time-sampling technique permitted documentation of how much receptive language in Spanish the baby had indeed acquired by one year from his father's daily conversational ritual (Friedlander *et al.*, 1972).

Increasing male involvement in researches and in children's lives

Males can be crucial as attachment figures and teachers for young children. However, *recruiting techniques* require creativity and ingenuity to enlist men into participation in early childhood settings or into research projects on fathering. By sitting for hours in free clinics for pregnant women in low-income neighborhoods, researchers were able to persuade unwed teens to enlist their male partners (who would become first-time fathers) into a program to teach young men in small groups, over several sessions, about infant and child development (Pfannenstiel & Honig, 1995). Half of the men were randomly assigned to a control group that was offered the program later on. Fathers were videotaped with their infants after the birth of the baby. The women were eager to help recruit fathers-to-be. Many expressed that this would be a way to keep the men involved in their lives. Clinical insights from this work were illuminating. Even when assigned randomly to the program group, some young men were dissuaded from participating because they were already intimate with a new partner and did not want anything to do with the baby soon to be born to the former girlfriend. Some of the fathers were talked into dropping out of the program by men in their workplace. Their buddies at work ridiculed the idea of the program by assuring the fathers that 'learning about babies is for girls and not for men!'

Recruiting *volunteers from high school and college classes* could increase the participation of men in ECE settings. This would serve to enhance and enrich the experiences both of young children and the young men who will be fathers someday.

Torelli (2008) urges that early administrators 'actively seek out men as caregivers and teachers. If you are not able to find fully qualified men, you should hire males as assistants and support their professional development so they can eventually become teachers ... Do you have a male cook or bus driver for your program? Invite them in the classroom' (p. 4).

Cunningham (1998) notes that the challenge is:

> How to *sell* men on the idea of volunteering. The question to think through is one of *What would a man get out of volunteering?* Or, if you are contacting an institution, *How would a high school or college benefit from having a male student volunteer with young children?* (p. 21)

As a consultant for a childcare center, I was once asked what could be done for an infant who had been crying and upset for over a month since enrollment despite staff efforts at comforting the child. The family was from China. I asked a Mandarin-speaking young man enrolled in one of our Child Development classes to go and volunteer in the center to hold the baby and talk to her in Mandarin for a few hours a few times a week. His loving reassuring words in Mandarin while tenderly holding her in his arms helped the baby become calmer and she was able to adjust to the center without further distress. Brainstorming how to provide *internship course credits for males* to work in ECE settings is important in order to increase male volunteer participation in childcare. Tables and booths staffed by current center volunteers, or by males enrolled in ECE courses, can be set up at high school and college events such as beginning semester Open House gatherings, or during school festivals or job fairs.

Senior Citizens centers are a good place to recruit retired grandfathers who could volunteer a few hours each week to spend with a preschooler in a center, particularly if transportation can be provided. Grandfathers spending intimate quality time one-on-one with a young child might be particularly felicitous for a child with no male role models in the family.

Ask fathers to help in projects requiring carpenter or building skills

To ensure that programming to increase positive father involvement is successful, it is important to ask fathers to explain their interests, wishes, priorities, and program offerings they would really like to attend. Enlisting dads' help in school painting or repair projects is another way to make fathers feel useful and in a more comfortable role in the center. One childcare facility was cited by the licensing agency for a broken slide outdoors. The children were then forbidden to play outdoors, and there were no funds to hire someone to take down that large piece of equipment. Several of the fathers found it an enjoyable cooperative activity to take down the large slide. They also felt satisfaction that the children could now once again use the outdoor space, even though that particular piece of play equipment was no longer available, until funds could be raised for a replacement.

Express appreciation for father participation

Fathers are only human in enjoying when they are asked courteously for help. 'Please' and 'Thank you' are important words for preschoolers to learn! Expressing genuine appreciation when fathers pitch in and provide services is a positive gesture that may lead to more paternal involvement in other classroom activities. A father might volunteer to come in and play guitar for a singing circle session. At the Children's Center in Syracuse, the teachers needed a solid wooden top for the ring stack set. They wanted to see whether toddlers would notice and reject that piece as not having the hole, which the other pieces had, and which is necessary if a piece is to fit over the ring stack pole. A father kindly volunteered to make a wooden plug. He sanded and smoothed the piece in his shop at home. The caregivers wrote him a special 'Thank you' note explaining about Piagetian spatial learning and how helpful he had been to contribute to making the toy more useful for their teaching work with the toddlers.

Ask already involved fathers for their ideas

Involved fathers can be enlisted to suggest ways to involve disengaged fathers. Brainstorm with small groups of involved fathers and elicit the creative suggestions they generate in order to 'lure' non-involved fathers into new activities, such as daily reading with their preschoolers, or participation in the centers their young children attend. One Head Start father (Rice, 2008), now on the Parent Advisory Board of the program where his child is enrolled, smiled as he recounted that he first became involved when his child's preschool program had a Poker Night just for dads! He also explained that he became ever more comfortable and involved as he came to know more of the fathers of his children's playmates in the center.

Other fathers, who work long hours away from home, report that they much prefer planned activities that *include* their wives and children, rather than activities that are exclusively men's programs. Fathers have different needs. Programs need to ask fathers for their ideas and craft a variety of program plans to increase father participation in the child's school world. When asked, fathers may of course suggest ideas quite different from those of mothers. In one EHS Center, the fathers designed a pizza party and also designed gift cards to be sent out to deserving fathers participating in program. The mothers, however, elected to dress up and go together for a night out at a restaurant. Berger (1998) offers more suggestions to involve fathers in early childhood programs:

- Promote partnerships between fathers. Match up new dads with current participants and form peer support groups.
- Provide fathers with information on child development. Teach them techniques for teaching sons *and* daughters of all ages.
- Make it easy for fathers to attend. Have flexible schedules. Provide or pay for transportation, and offer childcare.
- Offer life skills training. Teach classes on parenting relationships, anger management, and leadership.

- Help identify the abilities and needs of fathers. Provide literacy, job training, and employment opportunities, information, and referrals.
- Have men in leadership roles of the program.
- Promote tolerance. Encourage cultural diversity and acknowledge the important roles of mothers.
- Teach standards and accountability for fatherhood. Let dads know there are rights, responsibilities, resources and rewards ('four Rs of Fatherhood') to being a good father.
- Listen and learn from fathers. Survey men for their ideas and interests, and let them know you value their opinions.
- Recognize all kinds of fathers—from teen dads, to men who serve as father figures, to incarcerated fathers; remember that all dads need support (p. 60). Nowadays, videos are available for staff training to increase paternal involvement.

The 2007 *KidSafety of America* catalog, for example, lists videos with titles such as: 'Getting Men Involved in Childcare, Education, and Social work'; 'Young Men as Fathers' (available also in Spanish); and 'Developing and Maintaining a Young Fatherhood program' (www.kidsafetystore.com).

Currently, more magazines are apt to print articles praising positive father involvement. More books are being written addressed specifically for fathers. More authors of parenting books address parents of *both* genders and include many photographs of fathers (not just of moms) of different ages and from different culture groups in loving interactions with infants and young children (Honig & Brophy, 1996).

Newspapers in today's world provide space for stories that praise positive fathering. US Senator Bill Bradley (1998) wrote a newspaper column entitled 'Being a good dad should be a man's top goal.' He began thus:

> The most important thing a man can do in his life is to be a good father. All else pales— money, honor, celebrity. Fame and fortune pass. But with a child, you leave something of yourself behind. If you don't take this opportunity to do your best by your sons and daughters, you fail them and you fail your own humanity. (p. D3)

Men working in the world of childcare and elementary education

The growing interest in men's roles as early childhood educators received a special boost during the May 2008 conference exclusively devoted to this topic in Honolulu. Sponsored by the World Forum Foundation and the Hawaii Association for the Education of Young children, this conference on Men in Early Childhood Education, included topics such as:

- Men in the lives of children, families, and society.
- Research on the impact of male involvement in ECE.
- Recruiting and training male teachers.
- Constraints to increasing male involvement and how to overcome them.
- Curriculum strategies with men in mind.

- Dealing with abuse fears and allegations.
- Realities of daily life for men in early childhood programs.

Barriers to male involvement in childcare

There are many barriers to increased male involvement in childcare and nurturance, whether in enriching the paternal parenting role or in attempting to increase gender equality in childcare staffing (Cameron *et al.*, 2000).

Achieving gender balance through increasing men's roles in ECE settings has not and will not be an easy task! In Europe, the ECE Children's Network on Childcare prepared a lengthy report on male providers in childcare after interviews with providers, psychologists, parents, and psychiatrists in several countries. The Report emphasized: 'Childcare services remain one of the most gender segregated occupations in the entire labour force' (Jensen, 1995, p. 5). The figures they report for Denmark, Sweden, Finland, Spain, Belgium and the UK show that far more than 90% of childcare staff in the countries studied is female. Indeed, the Network reported that the debate on men in childcare in the UK, where over 98% of workers in 1981 were female, has led to restrictions on men, for example, not to put children on laps, and not to change a nappy without a female employee being present. The Network reports that such restrictions plus a focus on male sexuality, as if some male pedagogs must be gay, creates a work atmosphere of constant suspicion and discomfort for men.

The Network set out to study advantages and disadvantages of men working in childcare. As a positive example: children see a male staff member taking part in cooking and housekeeping scenarios with the children, and this helps challenge children's accepted stereotyped images of male roles.

The Report addressed obstacles to more men being employed. They suggested effective strategies to increase the number of men providing childcare. With respect to the latter goal, the Network described the 1988 decision of the Equal Rights Board in the municipality of Gothenburg, Sweden, to open a childcare center where the same number of men and women would be employed. After one year, men and women working at this center reported that staff was unusually 'free of conflicts.' Some of the men felt the wages were far too low; but this complaint is universal in the field for women as well as men in the USA too!

Women pedagogs in this study perceived that the men were much more accepted in childcare than women are usually accepted in male-dominated workplaces. They also felt appreciation of what they termed their specific female ways of doing things. Yet they also reported that they adopted what they termed a male way of talking to one another without feeling the subordination some women feel when talking with male bosses. Some of the male workers reported being overprotected by women who would do some caregiving chores for a male worker even when it was his turn.

Some children without fathers in the home hunger for male nurturance. Yet, male pedagogs in this study reported feeling uncomfortable when children of single mothers wanted to call them 'Daddy.' One center in the UK solved this problem by having the children call the male worker 'nursery daddy.'

One positive effect when staff included male workers was that *fathers were willing to spend more time at the center because there were male workers*. Since programs struggle in their attempts to involve fathers, increasing the number of male staff may be one positive approach to encourage more fathers of enrolled children to become active and involved in their children's center. Another positive effect was that girls, even though they usually chose different games from boys, were more likely, in a center with male teachers, to broaden the scope of their activities to include more spatial games.

The Report on the gender-equal center in Sweden soberly concluded that men would not stay on in caregiving jobs 'without demanding higher wages and advancement and would not show the subordination, patience, and loyalty that have been characteristic of women' (p. 12).

Cultural barriers

Other countries and culture groups face an uphill battle to include more male workers due to *different cultural attitudes toward the work of ECE teachers*. When I visited a special school for training kindergarten teachers in China two decades ago, the young women were learning wonderful crafts, such as intricate paper cutting, and other skills to bring to the children in classrooms where they would be serving as teachers. I asked our male translator in puzzlement why there were no men in that institute. Puzzled as well, he promptly replied: 'Why would a man want to become a kindergarten teacher?' Writing in the Beijing Review more recently, Hui (1997) reported that he was told ' No, we don't have male teachers nor do other kindergartens in Beijing.' However, in 1996, he reported that 49 men in the Shanghai No. 2 Preschool Teachers' School graduated to become kindergarten teachers. They are teaching the children more physical games, such as skating, as well as photography and Go. One director remarked 'they bring more vitality to the kindergarten.' (p. 22). It will be fascinating to see whether in the future China promotes more gender equity in the field of early childhood education.

The Sheffield Children's Centre in England has had a policy of recruiting male workers since 1985 and actively sought to make known its gender principles, policies, and practices to the wider community by means of the literature circulated in 12 different languages, by public meetings and discussion, direct targeting of men's groups, radio discussions and training events (Meleady, 1998). Following its early successes in hiring, recruitment later proved difficult with particular cultures— Somali, Arabic, and Pakistani communities:

> During meetings with male elders of the Somali community, the elders expressed the view that men caring for children was against the laws of nature and gave an example of how lions do not care for their young. Male staff from the Sheffield Centre responded to this with a description of Emperor Penguins. Following several meetings and awareness-raising sessions, a clear movement in perception became apparent and some Somali men were keen to pursue things ... [After] childcare training sessions and practical work experience, they became Centre workers—both unit and home-based. (p. 228)

Barriers due to sexual anxieties and suspicions

Williams (1993) interviewed men in traditionally female positions, such as teachers of the young or nurses. Some men felt they were in a dangerous position as single men working in elementary schools. They felt fearful about giving special attention to the children, particularly if a child was a female. A fourth-grade teacher said that because of possible misinterpretations, he would never give a child a hug!

> The men sensed others' conflicting definitions of the male role itself: the disciplinarian surrogate father engaged in 'unfeminine' activities, or the feminine, nurturing, empathic companion of children. The men in this study were forced to steer a course between these two equally dangerous extremes, either of which could result in suspicion and ultimate dismissal ... The need for male role models in early childhood education presents a series of dilemmas for male teachers. Conforming too closely to traditional definitions of masculinity again raises doubts about men's competence as teachers, while emphasizing nurturance and sensitivity opens men to the charges of effeminacy, or even worse. (p. 126)

Some of the men encountered people who considered them 'sexually suspect if they are employed in these "feminine" occupations either because they do or they do not conform to stereotypical masculine characteristics' (Williams, 1995, p. 108). Male workers reported using several emotional and practical 'distancing' strategies, such as focusing on certain technical or prestigious elements of their job when talking with outsiders, or seeing their current job as laying the groundwork for future jobs that would be more prestigious, such as working in a high school rather than with young children in elementary school, or going further in their education in order to become an administrator. One man reflected: 'The more I think about it, I'm sure that's a large part of why I wound up in administration. It's okay for a man to do the administration' (p. 136). Williams considers moving toward administration rather than providing direct childcare as one way that men can 'distance' themselves from women and carve out a masculine niche for themselves.

Interest in how to resolve some of the above issues successfully has increased in the past decades. In England, in 1998, Owen *et al.* published the proceedings of a seminar held in Henley on Thames on men as workers in services for young children. In the USA, a national study of attitudes toward male workers in ECE settings was carried out with 1000 early childhood professional workers randomly selected from the membership of the National Association for the Education of Young Children (Robinson *et al.*, 1984). Ninety percent of the sample of female and male teachers either disagreed or strongly disagreed with the item: 'Women are better suited by nature than men to work with preschool children.' Over 80% of teachers disagreed or strongly disagreed with the item: 'Many male preschool teachers tend to be effeminate.' Interestingly, 9.5% of male teachers agreed with this item.

No males but about 3% of female teachers agreed with the item: 'It is difficult to accept male preschool teachers because they are doing a woman's job.'

Almost one-fifth of male respondents and 13% of the women agreed with the item: 'Greater sensitivity and greater ability to nurture children tend to make women better suited than men for preschool teaching.' Most of the responses revealed similar views, regardless of respondent gender, about the capability and role of male preschool teachers and a lack of polarity of attitudes between men and women. The problem of stereotyping and prejudice against male educators with young children certainly exists among some parents and providers, but these data are encouraging in indicating that such prejudices are far less prevalent among some workers affiliated with early childhood organizations than has been assumed.

Myths about men in early childcare

Nelson (2004) has directly tackled some of the *myths* about why so few men work with young children and the stereotypes about men who do this work. One myth is that men won't work with young children because the wages are low. He points out that the U.S. Bureau of Labor Statistics reports men work in many low-paying jobs in the food industry, and in seasonal and temporary work. They are accepted in those settings and a critical point is that *other men are also working* in those settings. Thus it may be necessary to *hire a number of men in an ECE setting for other men to feel comfortable* in the job. Nelson points out that in the USA only 18.3% of elementary school teachers are men compared with 44.8% of secondary school teachers, yet union rules require that the salaries are the same!

Another *myth* is that men do not apply for ECE jobs. One survey in Ohio (Masterson, 1992) found that although Center directors hired women without degrees, they would not hire a man without an early childhood degree.

Another *myth* is that men who teach young children are gay. Male teachers are a diverse group. There are no data that provide evidence for the numbers of female or male childcare providers and ECE teachers who are straight, bisexual, or gay. Another *myth* is that men are more likely to leave the early childhood profession because of low wages. Women as well as men are likely to look for jobs that pay higher wages than childcare. Turnover rates in some facilities with only female teachers are over 40% annually in the USA.

Since childcare wages are low, men supporting families often face strong pressure to go into administration and move 'up' from the classroom, in order to earn increased wages. At the Children's Center in Syracuse, NY, one of the toddlers' most beloved teachers who created imaginative activities and had infinite patience with the children in his group, felt forced by economic necessity to leave our center and take a teaching position in elementary school (where salaries were higher) when his wife became pregnant with their third child.

Challenges and changes

Despite brave predictions that the percentages of men caring for and teaching young children in Western countries would be substantially increased in twenty-first century schools and nurseries, there is still a struggle to achieve gender equity. Politically, nations do not set a high priority on encouraging more positive and intimately engaged fathering interactions in families. There is still a long road to travel toward the goal of encouraging more men to participate in elementary classrooms and care centers with young children and to *stay* in the profession.

On a more promising note, more program descriptions are currently available that address the issue of how to recruit men for early childhood programs. Innovative strategies have been tried and provide a hopeful outlook. For example, Parents in Head Start's Community Action, in Minneapolis, redefined the role of the bus driver. They recruited their 54 Head Start bus drivers to become part of the ECE program and used this core of men to recruit other fathers. The drivers attend all educational staff meetings and also work one hour or more in the classroom (Levine *et al.*, 1993).

The rewards of those who choose to become early childhood care providers and teachers are eloquently expressed by McCartney (2007), a male teacher in the predominantly female world of early childhood. He reflected that:

> To become a better teacher I had to listen to children, respect them as individuals, question what I was doing, change my practices, and learn to be understanding and compassionate in my interactions with them. I had to take charge of my own professional growth and seek opportunities to further my understanding of early childhood development. ... I recently ran into a former parent. ... Eight or nine years ago, when her child came into my 2nd grade class, he was emotionally needy, unsure of himself, never a risk-taker, and dealing with family problems ... I remember treating him with compassion, care, and understanding ... [His mother] took my breath away when she said he wouldn't be where he is now (a self-assured young man) without my help and thanked me for being there for her son when he needed a strong male role model. ... Some children need a male teacher, but all children need a teacher that cares deeply about them. (p. 4)

This teacher so eloquently expresses the rewards for men as *persons* as well as teachers when they engage in the nurture and education of young children. Hopefully, more men will find the deep satisfactions in personal growth in work with young children.

Hopefully, too, society will reflect on this all-important work and choose to recompense more fairly those men as well as women who choose to serve as teachers and nurturers engaged in schools and childcare centers in the admirable adventure of actively and sensitively working to help young children flourish as learners and as kind and caring persons.

References

Administration for Children and Families (2006) *Head Start family and child experiences survey (FACES)* (Washington, DC, ACF).

Belsky, J. & Rovine, M. (1988) Nonmaternal care in the first year of life and security of infant-parent attachment, *Child Development*, 59, 157–167.

Berger, E. H. (1998) Don't shut fathers out, *Early Childhood Education Journal*, 26(1), 57–61.

Biller, H. (1970) Father absence and the personality development of the male child, *Developmental Psychology*, 2, 181–201.

Boller, K., Bradley, R., Cabrera, N. *et al.* (2006) The early head start father studies: design, data collection, and summary of father presence in the lives of infants and toddlers, *Parenting: Science and Practice*, 6(2, 3), 117–144.

Bonney, J. F., Kelley, M. L. & Levant, R. F. (1999) A model of fathers' behavioral involvement in child care in dual-earner families, *Journal of Family Psychology*, 113(3), 401–415.

Bradley, B. (1998, June 21) Being a good dad should be a man's top goal, *Syracuse Herald American*, p. D3.

Cameron, C., Moss, P. & Owen, C. (2000) *Men in the nursery: gender and caring work* (London, Paul Chapman).

Chase-Lansdale, P. L. & Owen, M. T. (1987) Maternal employment in a family context: effects on infant-mother and infant-father attachments, *Child Development*, 58, 1505–1512.

Cox, M. J., Owen, M. T., Henderson, V. K. & Margand, N. A. (1992) Prediction of infant-father and infant-mother attachment, *Developmental Psychology*, 28, 474–483.

Cowan, P. A., Cohn, D. A., Cowan, C. P. & Pearson, J. L. (1996) Parents' attachment histories and children's externalizing and internalizing behaviors: exploring family systems models of linkage, *Journal of Consulting and Clinical Psychology*, 64, 53–64.

Cunningham, B. (1998, September) Recruiting male volunteers to build staff diversity, *Child Care Information Exchange*, pp. 20–22.

Elder, G. H., Jr. (1974) *Children of the great depression* (Chicago, IL, University of Chicago Press).

Federal Interagency Forum on Child and Family Statistics (1998) *Nurturing fatherhood: improving data and research on male fertility, family formation and fatherhood* (Washington, DC, Author).

Fitzgerald, H. E., McKelvey, L. M., Schiffman, R. F. & Montanez, M. (2006) Exposure of low-income families and their children to neighborhood violence and paternal antisocial behaviors, *Parenting: Science and Practice*, 6(2, 3), 243–271.

Friedlander, B. Z., Jacobs, A. C., Davis, B. B. & Wetstone, H. S. (1972) A time-sampling analysis of infants/natural language environments in the home, *Child Development*, 43(3), 730–740.

Furstenberg, F. F., Jr., Morgan, S. P. & Allison, P. D. (1987) Paternal participation and child well-being after marital dissolution, *American Sociological Review*, 52, 695–701.

Grych, J. H. & Clark, R. (1999) Maternal employment and development of the father-infant relationship in the first year, *Developmental Psychology*, 35(4), 893–903.

Hewlitt, B. S. (2004) Fathers in forager, farmer, and pastoral cultures, in: M. E. Lamb (Ed.) *The role of the father in child development* (4th edn) (Hoboken, NJ, John Wiley), 182–195.

Honig, A. S. (1979) *Parent involvement in early childhood education* (Washington, DC, National Association for the Education of Young Children).

Honig, A. S. (1996) *Behavior guidance with infants and toddlers from birth to three years* (Little Rock, AR, Southern Early Childhood Education Association).

Honig, A. S. (2002). *Secure relationships: nurturing infant/toddler attachment in early care settings* (Washington, DC, National Association for the Education of Young Children).

Honig, A. S. & Brophy, H. (1996) *Talking with your baby: family as the first school* (Syracuse, NY, Syracuse University Press).

Honig, A. S. & Matsushita, W. (in preparation) *Mother and father perceptions of self and spousal degree of involvement in care activities with young children* (Syracuse University).

Honig, A. S. & Mayne, G. (1982) Black fathering in three social-class groups, *Ethnic Groups*, 4, 229–238.

Hui, W. (1997, January 20–26) Male kindergarteners appear and are loved, *Beijing Review*, pp. 22–23.

Hwang, C. P. (1986) Behavior of Swedish primary and secondary caretaking fathers in relation to mother's presence, *Developmental Psychology*, 22(6), 749–751.

Jensen, J. J. (1995) *Men as workers in childcare services* (London, European Commission Network on Childcare and other Measures to Reconcile Employment and Family Responsibilities).

Jung, K. & Honig, A. S. (2001) Intergenerational comparisons of paternal Korean child rearing practices and attitudes: a cross-cultural study, *International Journal of Early Childhood Education*, 7, 29–46.

Kelly, S. J. (1998) Men as childcare workers: are the risks worth the benefits? in: C. Owen, C. Cameron & P. Moss (Eds) *Men as workers in services for young children: issues of a mixed gender workforce*. Proceedings of a seminar held at Henley on Thames, 29–31 May 1997 (London, Institute of Education), 154–181.

Lamb, M. E. (2002) Nonresidential fathers and their children, in: C. S. Tamis-LeMonda & N. Cabrera (Eds) *Handbook of father involvement. Multidisciplinary perspectives* (Mahwah, NJ, Lawrence Erlbaum).

Lamb, M. E. (Ed.) (2004) *The role of the father in child development* (4th edn) (Hoboken, NJ, John Wiley).

Lamb, M. E. & Tamis-Lemonda, C. S. (2004) The role of the father in child development: an introduction, in: M. E. Lamb (Ed.) *The role of the father in child development* (4th edn) (Hoboken, NJ, John Wiley), 1–31.

Levine, J. A., Murphy, D. T. & Wilson, S. (1993) *Getting men involved: strategies for early childhood programs* (New York, Scholastic).

Maier, E. H. & Lachman, M. E. (2000) Consequences of early parental loss and separation for health and well-being in mid life, *International Journal of Behavioral Development*, 24, 183–189.

Marsiglio, W., Day, R. D. & Lamb, M. E. (2000) Exploring fatherhood diversity: implications for conceptualizing father involvement, *Marriage and Family Review*, 29, 269–293.

Masterson, T. (1992) A survey: attitudes of directors toward men, in: B. G. Nelson & B. Sheppard (Eds) *Men in child care and elementary education: a handbook for administrators and educators*. Available online at: www.MenTeach.org.

McCartney, M. (2007, Fall). Wanted: male teachers, *NYSAEYC Reporter*, pp. 1, 4.

McKeown, K., Ferguson, H. & Rooney, D. (1998) *Changing fathers?* (Cork, Ireland, Collins).

McLanahan, S. & Carlson, M. S. (2004) Fathers in fragile families, in: M. D. Lamb (Ed.) *The role of the father in child development* (4th edn) (Hoboken, NJ, John Wiley), 368–396.

Meleady, C. (1998). The Sheffield Children's Centre's experience of recruiting and training men to work in services for young children, in: C. Owen, C. Cameron & P. Moss (Eds) *Men as workers in services for young children: issues of a mixed gender workforce*. Proceedings of a seminar held at Henley on Thames, 29–31 May 1997 (London, Institute of Education), 225–233.

Nelson, B. G. (2004, November/December) Myths about men who work with young children, *Child Care Information Exchange*, 16–18.

Nelson, T. J., Clampet-Lundquist, S. & Edin, K. (2002) Sustaining fragile fatherhood. Father involvement in low-income, non-custodial African-American fathers in Philadelphia, in: C. S. Tamis-LeMonda & N. Cabrera (Eds) *Handbook of father involvement. Multidisciplinary perspectives* (Mahwah, NJ, Lawrence Erlbaum), 525–553.

Owen, C., Cameron, C. & Moss, P. (Eds) (1998). *Men as workers in services for young children: issues of a mixed gender workforce*. Proceedings of a seminar held at Henley on Thames, 29–31 May 1997 (London, Institute of Education).

Palkovitz, R. (2002) Involved fathering and child development: advancing our understanding of good fathering, in: C. S. Tamis-LeMonda & N. Cabrera (Eds) *Handbook of father involvement. Multidisciplinary perspectives* (Mahwah, NJ, Lawrence Erlbaum), 119–140.

Parke, R. D. & Brott, A. A. (1999) *Throwaway kids: the myths and barriers that keep men from being the fathers they want to be* (Boston, MA, Houghton Mifflin).

Pfannenstiel, A. & Honig, A. S. (1995). Effects of a prenatal 'Information and Insights about Infants' program on the knowledge base of first time, low-education fathers one month post-natally, *Early Child Development and Care*, 111, 87–105.

Phelps, A. (2008) What makes a great dad? *American baby*, LXX(6), 87.

Piburn, D. E. (2006, March/April) Gender equality for a new generation: expect male involvement, *Child Care Information Exchange*, pp. 18–22.

Pleck, J. H. (1997) Paternal involvement: levels, sources, and consequences, in: M. E. Lamb (Ed.) *The role of the father in child development* (3rd edn) (New York, Wiley), 66–103.

Raikes, H. A. & Bellotti, J. (2006) Two studies of father involvement in Early Head Start Programs: a national survey and a demonstration program evaluation, *Parenting: Science and Practice*, 6(2, 3), 229–242.

Rice, D. (2008). Roundtable: parenting and family outcomes in Head Start and Early Head Start, in: B. Allen (Chair) *Creating connections: program of the Head Start's Ninth Annual Research Conference*, Washington, DC, 23–25 June.

Robinson, B. E., Skeen, P. & Coleman, T. M. (1984) Professionals' attitudes toward men in early childhood education. A national study, *Children and Youth Services*, 6(2), 101–113.

Ryan, R. M., Martin, A. & Brookes-Gunn, J. (2006) Is one good parent good enough? Patterns of mother and father parenting and child cognitive outcomes at 24 and 36 months, *Parenting: Science and Practice*, 6(2, 3), 211–228.

Saey, T. H. (2008, March 29). Dad's hidden influence, *Science News*, pp. 200–201.

Steele, H., Steele, M. & Fonagy, P. (1996) Associations among attachment classification of mother, fathers, and their infants, *Child Development*, 15, 43–65.

Summers, J. A., Boller, K., Schiffman, R. F. & Raikes, H. H. (2006) The meaning of good fatherhood: low-income fathers' social constructions of their roles, *Parenting: Science and Practice*, 6(2, 3), 145–166.

Tamis-LeMonda, C. S. & Cabrera, N. (Eds) (2002) *Handbook of father involvement. Multidisciplinary perspectives* (Mahwah, NJ, Lawrence Erlbaum).

Tannen, D. (2001) *You just don't understand. Women and men in conversations* (New York, Morrow).

Torelli, L. (2008, March 28). Quality childcare. The missing element—men, *Child Care Information Exchange*. Available online at: http://www.spacesforchildren.com.men.html

Turbiville, V. P., Umbarger, G. T. & Guthrie, A. C. (2000) Fathers' involvement in programs for young children, *Young Children*, 55(4), 74–79.

Warin, J. (2006) Heavy-metal Humpty Dumpty: dissonant masculinities within the context of the nursery, *Gender and Education*, 18(5), 523–537.

Williams, C. L. (1993) *Doing 'Women's work': men in nontraditional occupations* (London, Sage).

Williams, C. L. (Ed.) (1995) *Still a man's world. Men who do women's work* (Berkeley, CA, University of California Press).

Yi, S. H. (1993) Transformation of child socialization in Korean culture, *Early Child Development and Care*, 85, 17–24.

Constructing identities: perceptions and experiences of male primary headteachers

Deborah Jones
Brunel University, UK

Background

The current context

The current context depicts a crisis in the recruitment of headteachers which is predicted to get worse. Indeed, between 2009 and 2011 there will be a critical short-age of headteachers (Maunder & Warren, 2008). A recent survey notes that 56% of heads are expected to retire in the next four years, the corollary of which is that there exists an urgent need to recruit 10,000 new headteachers (GTC, 2008). Newspaper reports reflect the general public concern over the developing crisis, for example: 'Report highlights crisis in headteacher recruitment' (MacLeod, 2007) and '10,000 heads to leave red tape behind' (Milne & Bloom, 2008). As the latter report notes, key to the crisis is the increased administrative responsibilities which have become integral to headteacher roles in recent years.

Many primary headteachers it appears are experiencing high levels of stress and a constantly increasing workload. In 2002, The National College for School Leadership (NCSL) was established to provide and coordinate professional leadership and in so doing to address in part the headteacher shortage. In their recent advice to the Secretary of State on primary leadership they assert that:

> Primary heads are under increasing pressure from an unprecedented mix of high levels of devolved responsibility, sharp accountability structures, and radical changes in the way schools interact with other services and their communities ... (they) deal with too many operational issues and administrative tasks. (2007, p. 4)

Further, the guidance notes that the small size of many primary schools makes it difficult to institute distributed leadership, so placing unnecessary strain on individual headteachers.

The General Teaching Council (GTC) (2008) acknowledges that only 4% of teachers are considering becoming heads in the next five years. A survey into teacher workload (MORI, 2006) found that top reasons for not pursuing headship among middle managers and deputies were as follows: stress; personal commitments; less pupil contact, less teaching involvement; administrative demands; inspection and accountability. Specifically then, 70% of middle leaders and 43% of deputies had no desire to become heads.

Gender factors

In addition, there are gender related issues. The numbers of male headteachers are over represented across all phases and are vastly disproportionate. In the primary sector, although 83% of teachers are women, only 62% are heads (Department for Education and Skills [DfES], 2005). Teaching in the primary sector has become feminised while leadership in this context has become masculinised (Blount, 1999). Historical discourses come into play in this regard. One difficulty that men face in entering the profession is that they are perceived as doing 'women's work'. The teaching of young children in particular is associated with women for two main reasons: first, because caring is perceived as essentially a female quality, the construction of 'mother' being perceive as akin to the social construction of 'teacher' (Noddings, 2005) and secondly, as a result of the history of gendered skewed job occupation.

There is clear evidence of the glass elevator operating within the context of primary education (Martin, 1991). Here, men in female-dominated organisations earn more and are promoted faster than their female counterparts (Snyder, 2008). 'Men take their gender privilege with them when they enter predominantly female occupations'

(Williams, 1992, p. 6). Men's clubs are clearly in evidence within primary teaching. Male students are aware that they will be fast-tracked and in part, as a result of the public discourse it becomes both more acceptable and more preferable for them to occupy management positions (Jones, 2007). This reflects international trends where statistics 'verify the persistent dominance of White males in school leadership roles' (Rusch & Marshall, 2006, p. 230).

Given the current pressures on heads in general but the greater number of males in the field, what then are the perceptions and experiences of male headteachers within the primary context? How do male headteachers construct their identities and how does their awareness of wider discourses in this regard impact on their working lives?

The study

A small scale research project was undertaken to investigate male and female head-teachers' perceptions and experiences of working in the early years of schooling. A post-structuralist approach was taken, as it is concerned with the production of iden-tities, and with how identities change within various contexts (Kenway, 1994). Approaching research from this position enabled reflection on multiple practices in schools. It allowed a focus on how identities of male and female headteachers are co-constructed within the school context. Adopting this stance informed an analysis of power relations as they operated in and around the school context and the impact that had on identity (Francis, 1996).

A key concept drawn from post-structuralism is discourse and this research focuses on how institutions and those working within them are affected and produced by wider ideological discourses. A post-structuralist approach, then, facilitates an understanding of meaning-making processes and connections between local and historical discourses (Mauthner & Hey, 1999). This research attempts to breakdown the dominant discourses and examine the complexities of their produc-tion and acceptance.

Semi-structured interviews were undertaken with a cross section of 10 male head-teachers and 10 female headteachers. The focus in this article will be on the male headteachers.

Ten different schools were selected from four different local authorities. Of these were six primary schools (4–11) of which four included nursery provision, two junior schools (7–11), one infant nursery school (3–7) and one all through faith school (5–18). Schools were of various sizes and were placed in contexts where socio-economic factors differed considerably. The one common factor was that all schools worked in partnership with the University and all were used to taking students.

In each school the male headteacher was interviewed. Heads reflected a diversity of backgrounds and experience. The eldest was aged 64 and the youngest 32. Length of teaching experience ranged from 13 to 42 years, while length of time as a head ranged from one to 37 years. Regarding ethnic background nine were White-European and one was British South-Asian. Several had experience of working in countries other than the UK.

Six headteachers had begun teaching after completing their teaching qualifications which they had embarked upon straight after school, while four had joined the profession from other occupations. Of the latter group previous jobs included civil servant, optician, computing work and solicitor.

Semi-structured interviews of up to one hour were undertaken with individual men in order to elicit rich data (Lofland *et al.*, 2005). Analysis of interview transcripts revealed similar themes and patterns emerged. Integral to these patterns were major discourses concerning identity and power. Here, however the focus will be on the construction of male headteachers' identities. The next section will explore several influential discourses as they relate to male headteachers' identities. What follows will examine themes inherent in male headteachers' discourses as they reflect upon their roles and experiences within the early years contexts and consider the practice of identity construction. This research, then, attempts to explore the complexities of this process.

Constructing identities

The post-modern concept of identity asserts that there is a 'crisis of identity' which is undermining the security of both groups and individuals. Identities are neither fixed, stable nor permanent, but change according to the variety of cultural systems which present themselves, thus assuming different identities at different times. As Hall (2003) puts it: 'we are confronted by a bewildering, fleeting multiplicity of possible identities, any one of which we could identify with, at least temporarily' (p. 277).

Individuals operate across a range of different contexts, or 'fields' (Bourdieu, 1984) such as family, work and so on. Operating within these very different contexts may draw from us a range of different identities. We are governed by certain social expectations which result in us positioning ourselves, or being positioned according to the 'fields' of operation. Not only are we faced with a multiplicity of identities, but some may conflict and result in tensions for the individual (Curry-Johnson, 2001). There would appear to be ambiguity and often discomfort, not only over who, but also, over how, to be.

This is of particular relevance to any discussion of masculinities which depend upon culture and are shaped differently at different times (Berger *et al.*, 1995). So, it may be held, that what we are currently witnessing in contemporary society is a form of 'hybridised' masculinity, experienced and presented differently according to context. Indeed, Beynon (2002) describes this process as 'nothing less than the emergence of a more fluid, bricolage masculinity, the result of "channel hopping" across versions of the masculine' (p. 6). It is this view which characterises the post-modern man.

Integral to these processes are notions of power. So, practices which produce meaning involve relations of power. Individuals can neither be free from, nor operate outside of, the exercise of power (Foucault, 1984). It is diffuse, interwoven into society operates through networks and allows for the exploration of different discourses at different times. We are subject to certain discourses and have a certain amount of agency in deciding not only whether or not we will take them up, but also where exactly we will position ourselves. There has been significant debate concerning the process of reflexive modernisation, whereby individuals are no longer affiliated to traditional gender identities (Adkins, 2002). As a result of this loosening of identity, an autobiography of choice exists (Beck, 2001), whereby we can become who we want to be. Importantly, however, agency is constrained by the operation of various factors. Power structures operating within relations of class and gender, for example, may mean individuals do not exercise absolute choice over the discourses which eventually position them (Woodward, 2002, p. 39).

Within the following study, male headteachers discuss several differing identities which they construct for themselves and which they choose to inhabit. In addition, they are aware that various groups have the power to construct their identities in different ways. Different groups of people such as parents and governors also have a major role to play in this process of identity construction as they interact with men and exert their influence. This article will discuss different identities constructed by and for male headteachers and will argue that individuals may be limited as far as choice is concerned because of the power structures operating both within the primary school institution and in wider society.

The male primary headteacher: constructing identities

The expert

Male headteachers had a strong sense of their own abilities and in most cases an over-riding self-confidence: 'I hate to call it arrogance, but there's a self-confidence that I can do it'. In general they assumed the role of expert among their staff: 'I mean I hold the reigns pretty tightly … and it's not about my head being on the block, it's because I believe I'm right'.

Additionally, most male headteachers included that sense of being 'better than others' as a factor within their initial motivation for headship.

> I saw someone who was appointed to headship and I thought, with all due respect, I can offer as much if not so much more. Not trying to be arrogant but I didn't think it was a good appointment.

As this illustrates, most were disparaging in their comments about certain male teachers or heads they had observed and constructed themselves as 'other' in relation to them. There existed a commonly held notion of two extremes of men in primary schools, 'very rarely is there the middle ground'. It was acknowledged that there were some very good male teachers, but that these were 'the exception not generally the rule'. The following describes this view:

> the male teaching force in primary education … we're good at the extremes, so you're either very, very good, or you're not very good at all.

This exemplifies the process of binary construction whereby different identities may be construed as 'other', 'deviant' or outside of what is acceptable by the mainstream (Butler, 1993). In this way some individuals are relegated to outsider status or marginalised if they 'break the rules'. Male primary teachers are liable to be marginalised by other men in particular and society in general as they operate in a feminised world (Smedley, 2007). What appears to be operating here is the 'othering' of inadequate males within the profession who do not measure up to hegemonic masculinity in terms of their capabilities to operate as 'expert leader'.

Male heads were anxious to distance themselves from such men who were described as 'incompetent', 'ineffective', 'useless' and who, in some cases, had come into teaching because 'they had failed other things in the past'. The male heads quite firmly placed themselves at the opposite end of the continuum as being both excellent and outstanding.

The role model

The majority of heads thought there should be more men working in primary education and all cited the need for role models as a main reason. There did not, however, appear to be much clarity as to what a male role model was. The discourse of 'common sense' appears to operate, that is, it is self-evident that males in primary contexts are a 'good thing'. Sargent (2001) supports the finding that this concept is uncritically embedded in the discourse of teachers. Some suggested that male role models are a good thing, simply because they are not female, so drawing upon notions of women as 'other', for example:

> A male head will just through his sheer demeanour present things in a slightly different way (to women).

Others cite balance as a reason for introducing more male role models, but again few could articulate why that would be beneficial. The notion of 'balance is interesting, suggesting "fairness" and equity'. Some did attempt to unpick this aspect and described the need for a 'stable male' or 'father figure' in children's lives. They were aware that some children, especially boys, viewed them as such.

The call to recruit more men into teaching, the fact that numbers of male heads in the primary sector are vastly disproportionate, fit with the public discourse surrounding the drive for more male role models. Presumably, the kind of role model desired would exhibit characteristics of hegemonic masculinity and instigate this in male pupils. The implications of this give cause for concern, not least because a feature of such masculinity is its dominance and subordination of other groups, both male and female (Connell, 2004). This was recognised by several heads in this study:

> I guess my disquiet is a lot of the male role models I've seen in primary schools are not good, and therefore it's counter productive. Um, so I think it would be wonderful to have some very positive role models ... but they are few and far between I think.

The situation is a complex one. Who decides what a 'good' role model is? Indeed an 'influx of conservative & uncritical men could simply reinforce more traditional patterns of gender relations' (Lingard & Douglas, 1999, p. 57). In some instances, heads made the point that their own perceptions of role models differed from views held in wider society:

> A positive male role model is ... someone who's ... empathetic to the needs of the children and brings a bit of creativity. He doesn't do a lot of shouting around and all that macho stuff.

Male heads were also very aware of their status as role model not only in relation to children, but also with regard to their staff, parents and governors:

> Governing bodies on the whole may prefer to appoint a man ... maybe it's about role models for staff and children.

The importance of being a role model who leads by example was also highlighted:

> I felt it was my role to prove myself, to prove that I could do the job, that I was worth whatever I was being paid, that I was worth the title and the role ... [A teacher was overheard to say] 'From the minute he got here [he] has not asked us to do anything he would not do himself'.

However, the difficulty remains that definitions of the male role model are not explicitly articulated within the public discourse where there appears to be no clear consensus as to what an effective male role model is. It appears that all male heads are open to stereotyping simply by virtue of being male. By definition this process is unthinking, identities being constructed for males which may be far removed from the qualities which they do, in fact, exhibit.

The authority figure/disciplinarian

Authority.   For male headteachers, there was a very real sense of enjoying the position of authority that came with the role: 'At the end of the day I like controlling what goes on'. This was a typical response. Male heads were aware of being propelled into leadership positions by groups within society and had realised usually from the start of their careers that their promotion chances were good:

> The stats in terms of headship, I suppose, reflect the partly the drive men feel. They feel there's a very good chance of them getting there, so they're driven by that, driven by ambition, driven by the need to be in charge.

There is a sense then in which identity is bound up with a sense of power and this is constantly reinforced to heads from a range of different groups, for example,

> I showed a prospective parent around and she said 'the school is the Head isn't it. It reflects your ambition, it reflects your philosophy, it reflects what you're all about'.

This illustrates the position held by some that the identity of the head is actually fused with that of the school—the ultimate signifier of authority.

Discipline.   The men in this study were aware of both parents and governors in particular, expressing preconceptions of the male head as firm disciplinarian.

> There is unfortunately a perspective within communities that a male head will provide more discipline within the school ... I think there are often quite a lot of parents who are happier, particularly the fathers in dealing with a male head. That's the sort of feedback I get.

This connects to the trend of male teachers being concentrated in the upper years of schooling and, together with the male head, being perceived as the main source of discipline (Beynon, 1989). In this way it appears, there is an attempt to mirror conventional masculinity (Connell, 2004).

The view that the preference of governing bodies was to appoint men and that this was tied up with the male role of disciplinarian was commonly held: 'Governing bodies tend to think a male figure has this certain something or would be better at discipline'. This notion that men are better at discipline than women is firmly embedded in the public discourse (Miller, 1997; Cammack & Phillips, 2002). Indeed, Johannesson (2004) found that women teachers in particular are familiar with this discourse but are, in fact, critical of it.

Status

Uncomfortable issues commonly emerged as men were conscious of perceptions of primary teaching and even headship as low status within the public discourse. One head described the changing views of his father in relation to career trajectory:

> Dad very much felt it wasn't a real career, it wasn't a proper job ... I don't think he saw it as a man's job ... because I wanted to do primary education that made it even worse, it was all female teachers. But, when I got to Deputy and when I got to this—he was proud.

Male heads were aware that the weight of society's views on men working with young children is negative. Implicit in their responses are notions of primary teaching as 'women's work' or low status:

> Very occasionally I get asked by people 'what do you do?' 'I'm a headteacher of a primary school' and then we go on to 'Are you hoping to become head of a secondary school one day?' as if it's somehow a promotion. I used to get—'you're only an infant teacher' I suppose it's about perceived status.

This is 'soft', female work, not in keeping with the 'harder' more 'macho' types of career. So men within primary school contexts have their masculinity called into question (Skelton, 2003). This end is perhaps the most innocuous, expressing the view that because they are in a feminised profession, they are not quite 'real men' and in some instances, not quite 'real heads'.

Therefore certain discourses may be catalysts for removing men from the classroom situation, propelling them towards roles seen as more fitting for men. Most male heads, from an early stage, viewed management positions as the obvious end point for their careers and had made strategic decisions to fast-track and enter better paid managerial positions. Yet, as is illustrated above even headship of primary schools is not perceived to carry the equivalent status of heads at secondary level. The view of work with young children as low status persists (Jones, 2007).

Nurturer

Closer involvement. There did, however, appear to be a disconnect between the perception of headteacher as distant disciplinarian prevalent in some sectors of society and the desire in several cases of male heads to assume a closer, warmer identity with both children and adults:

> The male headteacher in this country if you asked adults to describe it would be a figure of authority, fairly distant, behind a desk where discipline is what they get involved in ... I regret that distance ... I would like to have a warmth of relationship, ease with parents that I've seen in other countries, and that I see between some female heads and their parents ... It seems more relaxed.

Several male heads spoke of a desire to display greater affection with the children but were aware of the difficulties this may present.

Constraints

It appeared that male heads are aware of more serious scrutiny pertaining to their motivation and, in some instances, their masculinity

> There's a little lad who's six and he holds my hand in the playground. He hasn't got a dad and to him maybe I'm a dad figure ... we've got many children who could benefit from touch, but as a man I'm very, very careful ... I confine myself to a pat on the head or shoulder.

As evidenced in this study and others (Skelton, 2001; NFER, 2002), men in primary education are acutely aware of 'touch' discourses which contribute to their aspirations of moving into a managerial role or even leaving the profession (Foster, 1995). They are aware of accusations that may be levelled against them resulting in 'moral panic' arising within the public discourse. In several instances, they desired to show more affection but thought better of it: 'for your own protection you have to be careful'. All men who enter and stay in the profession have to deal with suspicion (Martino & Berrill, 2003) and may at certain points be perceived as 'high risk' (McWilliam & Jones, 2005). Male heads it appears, although cushioned to some extent by their managerial position, are not exempt from this.

Nurturing children

With regard to care, dominant forms of male heterosexuality are characterised by the need to avoid closeness in relationships and to fear emotions (Kimmel, 1994; Connell, 2005). Caring, on the other hand, may be perceived as the prerogative of women, who are widely held as being 'better for the job' and dominate the caring professions. Some feminist perspectives support the view that caring is a strength which is particular, although not exclusive to women (Noddings, 2005). It may also be maintained that men are capable of caring for young children, which may be regarded as uncommon, but nevertheless well within their capacities (King, 2005).

In the following statement the head is reflecting upon the impact of such discourses on his role:

> I feel you have to prove something ... That you can work with this age children and not necessarily be a woman and therefore have the intrinsic qualities of being a mother and, you know, be someone who can look after a child who has fallen over and hurt themselves. It is possible to do all those as a man.

Another head comments on the capabilities of men to be nurturers, which again is something that flies in the face of the dominant public discourse:

> I think society at large has got a very skewed view of what men in education are about, 'oh a man can't be responsible for a five- or six-year old', but men can set up such nurturing environments and have all the qualities that you wouldn't necessarily expect in a male role model.

As a result men are pushed towards the upper years of schooling where the pressure from society in this regard is not as great. Yet, another makes the point that he has 'a maternal and paternal instinct...' and that although the desire to work in the early years may be strong, men are made to feel less comfortable about operating in this sector. Nevertheless the role of nurturer formed a significant part of men's reflections and was not simply confined to their interaction with children. For most interviewed it extended to their relationships with their staff and was seen as central to their function as headteacher:

> It's as pleasing, as with children, to see staff who have come in as Newly Qualified Teachers, and you have nurtured them and they have developed and then they move on to deputy headships.

For these heads, their role as nurturer of both children and staff spawned a significant amount of satisfaction, pleasure and reward.

The family man

Several men acknowledged that the structure of society benefited them.

> The forces of family life are structured to help men ... when you look at the proportion of women who go on to become headteachers that's a clear one. The women are able to maybe manage being a classteacher and manage a family, but the demands of headship ...

They recognised that they owed a significant amount to partners who supported them in many ways freeing them up to be single-minded about their professional lives:

> Marrying a wife like mine is a very wise thing to do for anybody like me because you get extremely well fed and looked after ... she can do loads of things and I'm obsessive about one thing.

This is supported by a recent survey of headteachers where it was found that 'in three-quarters of the households of the men headteachers, their wives or partners take the major responsibility for all domestic matters' (Coleman, 2007, p. 390). However, most reflected on the cost of headship to their lives within the family:

> Um I think there have been times ... that my time spent with my son, when he was growing up was truncated by things ... it was impinged upon by my work.

The time factor was significant in that male heads noted that precious time with their families was given over to work in school often undertaking long hours or evening work: 'I've got a young son and I will barely see him this week'. This impacted not only on children, but also on partners. It affected not only the amount of time spent with them, but in some instances the quality of relationship:

> My partner would say that I was never quite the same after I became a head ... in that the main cost is the accountability thing ... you do consider things that are going on in the school in the holidays.

In some cases the costs of headship were even greater as one head reflects:

> Right OK, divorce. Yes without a doubt um ... being quite open and honest, the cost would be my marriage ... but my whole goal was you've got to be successful ... and when I talk about failure, that's the biggest failure of my life without a doubt. So the cost of being successful and putting time in and doing this, this and this, which at the time I did think was the right thing—wasn't.

Interestingly, in some instances it appeared that school had, to some extent, taken on the characteristics of family, as one head notes: 'It's almost like having your own children that sense of pride, that desire for them to do well'. Equally the relationship between heads and children was not devoid of significant emotion. This is reflected in the following observation:

> There is nothing more pleasurable than seeing children leave at the end of Year 6. You remember those children as little infants that came into the school so vulnerable ... you see them and think you're at the start of your adult life no and you've seen them flourish and it literally brings a tear to your eye, because, you know, it reminds you of what the job is all about, it's about developing children and preparing them for adult life.

The parallel between their role as head and parenting was frequently drawn: 'Some of these children need parenting—I'd like to take them home'. There is a sense in which the identity of family man finds expression in both home and work, but may offer differing levels of fulfilment in each.

Summary

For any male, working within the context of primary education, at headship level or as classteacher the situation is a complex one. Different identities are constructed for them by parents, governors and wider society. Many of the difficulties they encounter are related to perceptions of early years education as 'women's work'. As noted, certain feminist explanations of care (Noddings, 2005) have depicted women as better carers and thereby more suited to work with young children. In addition, biologism has been drawn upon, where, by virtue of their role as mothers, women are also held to be more appropriate for primary school teaching. These same epistemologies, however, of essential feminine nurturance have been used to devalue women's skills within institutions contributing to the low status and low pay of caring professions.

Further, men who attempt to take on caring roles, or indeed who operate in this context may be subject to the same denigration as women. Moreover, the public discourse is liable to construct them as objects of derision at worst or as not to be taken seriously at best. Men who enter the early years environment run the risk of becoming less than respectable. The identity of 'inadequate male' may be constructed for them.

For many male teachers, their initial years within the primary school can be fraught with uncertainty and discomfort. For them, a key factor in this process of establishing identity is that of identification, whereby male teachers position themselves in places constructed by discourses. There is, however, a limit to agency as they may be positioned in certain ways by discourses over which they have no control (Woodward, 2002). Discourses of male teachers as 'high risk', for example, cannot be ignored and men working with young children must somehow accommodate to the fact such discourses exist. Nevertheless, insecurity for men appears to be relatively short-lived, in part because of systems of power. So men are pushed into the upper years of schooling and are aware that they may be fast-tracked into leadership roles as evidenced by the disproportionate numbers of male heads in primary education. It is therefore difficult to see how selection of identity can work devoid of power. The propensity of governing bodies to view males a more suited to headship supports this (Coleman, 2007). Power, then, would appear to be interwoven into wider society, operating from many different points within it (Foucault, 1984). It operates through networks and allows for the exploration of different discourses at different times. The trajectory of the male teacher from student to headteacher is characterised by an awareness of power shifting between individuals, cutting across hierarchies and short-circuiting established stratas of authority (Jones, 2007).

Most of the heads in this study illustrated the concept of 'bricolage' masculinity (Beynon, 2002). They attempted to construct their identities through drawing upon a range of available masculinities (Haywood & Mac an Ghaill, 2003). They revealed elements of hegemonic masculinity, together with masculinities which were sensitive, caring and nurturing. It may appear then that becoming a headteacher with its distance from the 'messy' work on the ground goes some way to removing the stigma of 'inadequate male' and heads demonstrated a keenness to distance themselves from this particular identity.

They clearly enjoyed being 'in authority' and as men in leadership positions derive benefit from the 'patriarchal dividend' (Connell, 2005). This is evidenced in that they are not subject to the same slights as some male class-teachers. However, issues of status emerge as they compete against the discourse of primary head as subordinate to the secondary head. Nevertheless in contrast they assumed identities of the competent, efficient, powerful leader.

The man of authority better fits the characteristics of hegemonic masculinity, nevertheless the pressure on men to conform to the commonly held stereotype of 'distant head' presents difficulties for them and in some instances an acutely felt lack of integrity. The role of headship may be viewed as a double-edged sword. On the one hand, it functions to protect men from the denigration to which other male teachers are sometimes subject. On the other, it can operate to distance them from closer relationships which they frequently wish for, not only with children, but with parents and staff. Male heads are aware that they are constantly measured against the stereotype of hegemonic masculinity which brings both protection—through the demonstrations of power—and restriction in that they are limited in the conduct of relationships. As such, although rewarding, the role is characterised by complexity.

References

Adkins, L. (2002) *Revisions: gender and sexuality in late modernity* (Buckingham, Open University Press).

Beck, U. (2001) *World risk society* (Cambridge, Polity Press).

Berger, M. (1995) *Constructing masculinity* (New York, Routledge).

Beynon, J. (1989) *A school for men* (Milton Keynes, Open University Press).

Beynon, J. (2002) *Masculinities and culture* (Buckingham, Open University Press).

Blount, J. M. (1999) Manliness and the gendered construction of school administration in the USA, *International Journal of School Leadership in Education*, 2(2), 55–68.

Bourdieu, P. (1984) *Distinction: a social critique of the judgement of taste* (Cambridge, MA, Harvard University Press).

Butler, J. (1993) *Bodies that matter* (New York, Routledge).

Cammack, J. C. & Philips, D. K. (2002) Discourses and subjectivities of the gendered teacher, *Gender and Education*, 14, 123–133.

Coleman, M. (2007) Gender and educational leadership in England: a comparison of secondary headteachers' views over time, *School Leadership and Management*, 27(4), 383–399.

Connell, R. W. (2004) *Gender* (Cambridge, Polity Press).

Connell, R. W. (2005) *Masculinities* (Berkeley, CA, University of California Press).

Curry-Johnson, S. (2001) Weaving an identity tapestry, in: B. Findlen (Ed) *Listen-up: voices from the next feminist generation* (Seattle, WA, Seal Press), 51–58.

Department for Education and Skills (DfES) (2005) *Statistics of education: teachers.* (London, DfES).

Foster, T. (1995) You don't have to be female to survive on this course but it helps, *Redland Papers*, 3, 35–42.

Foucault, M. (1984) *The history of sexuality: an introduction* (vol. 1) (London, Penguin).

Francis, B. J. (1996) *Children's constructions of gender, power and adult occupation.* Unpublished Ph.D. thesis, University of North London.

General Teaching Council (GTC) (2008) *Survey of teachers 2007.* Available online at: http://www.gtce.org.uk/research/tsurvey/ (accessed 1 July 2008).

Hall, S. (2003) The question of cultural identity, in: S. Hall, D. Held, & T. McGrew (Eds) *Modernity and its futures* (Buckingham, Open University Press), 273–326.

Haywood, C. & Mac an Ghaill, M. (2003) *Men and masculinities* (Buckingham, Open University Press).

Johannesson, I. A. (2004) To teach boys and girls: a pro-feminist perspective on the boy's debate in Iceland, *Educational Review*, 56(1), 33–41.

Jones, D. (2007) Millennium man: constructing identities of male teachers in early years contexts, *Educational Review*, 59(2), 179–194.

Kenway, J. (1994) Making hope practical rather than despair convincing: feminist poststructuralism, gender reform and educational change, *British Journal of the Sociology of Education*, 15(2), 187–210.

Kimmel, M. S. (1994) Masculinity as homophobia: fear, shame, and silence in the construction of gender identity, in: H. Brod & M. Kaufman, (Eds) *Theorizing Masculinities* (Thousand Oaks, CA, Sage), 119–141.

King, J. R. (2005) *Uncommon caring: learning from men who teach young children* (New York, Teachers College Press).

Lingard, B. & Douglas, P. (1999) *Men engaging feminisms: pro-feminisms, backlashes and schooling* (Buckingham, Open University Press).

Lofland, J., Anderson, L., Snow, D. & Lofland, L. H. (2005) *Analysing social settings: a guide to qualitative observation & analysis* (Belmont, CA, Wadsworth).

MacLeod, D. (2007, August 31) Report highlights crisis in headteacher recruitment, *The Guardian*. Available online at: http://www.guardian.co.uk/education/2007/aug/31/schools.uk (accessed 13 March 2008).

Martin, L. (1991) *A report on the glass ceiling initiative* (Washington, DC, U.S. Department of Labour).

Martino, W. & Berrill, D. (2003) Boys, schooling and masculinities: interrogating the 'right' way to educate boys, *Education Review*, 55(2), 99–117.

Maunder, M. & Warren, E. (2008) *Is there still a glass ceiling?* (West Sussex, National Association of Headteachers).

Mauthner, M. & Hey, V. (1999) Researching girls: a poststructuralist approach, *Educational and Child Psychology*, 16(2), 67–84.

McWilliam, E. & Jones, A. (2005) An unprotected species? On teachers as risky subjects, *British Educational Research Journal*, 31(1), 109–120.

Miller, J. H. (1997) Gender issues embedded in the experience of student teaching: being treated like a sex object, *Journal of Teacher Education*, 48, 10–28.

Milne, J. & Bloom, A. (2008, February 1) 10,000 heads to leave red tape behind, *The TES*. Available online at: http://www.tes.co.uk/search/story/?story_id=2577563 (accessed 13 March 2008).

MORI (2006) *Teacher workload survey* (London, Author).

National College for School Leadership (NCSL) (2007) *Primary leadership: advice to the secretary of state* (Nottingham, Author).

NFER (2002) *Recruitment to and retention on initial teacher training: a systematic review* (Berkshire, Author).

Noddings, N. (2005) *The challenge to care in schools: an alternative approach to education* (New York, Teachers College Press).

Rusch, E. & Marshall, C. (2006) Gender filters and leadership: plotting a course to equity, *International Journal of Leadership in Education*, 9(3), 229–250.

Sargent, P. (2001) *Real men or real teachers? Contradictions in the lives of men elementary school teachers* (Harriman, TN, Men's Studies Press).

Skelton, C. (2001) *Schooling the boys: masculinities and primary education* (Buckingham, Open University Press).

Skelton, C. (2003) Male primary teachers and perceptions of masculinity, *Education Review*, 55(2), 195–210.

Smedley, S. (2007) Learning to be a primary school teacher: reading one man's story, *Gender and Education*, 19(3), 369–385.

Snyder, K. A. (2008) Revisiting the glass escalator: the case of gender segregation in a female dominated occupation, *Social Problems*, 55(2), 271–299.

Williams, C. (1992) The glass escalator: hidden advantages fro men in the female professions, *Social Problems*, 39, 253–267.

Woodward, K. (Ed) (2002) *Identity and difference: culture, media and identities* (London, Sage).

Gender and professionalism: a critical analysis of overt and covert curricula

Michel Vandenbroeck and Jan Peeters

Gent University, Belgium

Gender segregation

Since many decades, scholars in the field of early childhood education deplore the gender segregation in the caring professions. Since the famous study of Lamb (1975), there is a growing consensus that the presence of men as carers would benefit the child. In the early 1980s already, the European Union started a first Gender Equality programme (Moss, 1996) and four years later, the European Commission Childcare Network was launched. One of its three actions was focused on 'Men as Carers', aiming to attract more men in the early childhood workforce (Moss, 1996). In 1992, the Council of Ministers of the European Union (1992) issued the Recommendations on Childcare, stating (Article 6) that 'member states commit themselves to promote

and encourage, with due respect for the freedom of the individual, increased participation by men'. Experts agreed on the necessity to attract more men in the child care
workforce. It was argued that this may serve as a role model for fathers to take up a
more active role in their families by creating a more gender-neutral caring culture. A
second equally important reason was that children in services for young children
would benefit from the confrontation with different role models and this in turn may
affect their gender socialisation. Consequently, the altered gender socialisation may
enhance more equal gender roles in future generations (European Commission
Childcare Network, 1993). When, in 1995, the European Commission published its
Forty Quality Targets in Services for Young Children, target 29 stipulated explicitly
that by 2005, 20% of the caring professionals should be male (Moss, 1995).
However, little progress has been made since. In 1995, Denmark had the highest
percentage of men in child care: 5%, followed by Finland (4%) and Sweden (3%).
The UK reached only 2% men and Flanders 1.5% in centre-based care and 0.5% in
home-based care (Jensen, 1998). In the last years, there are additional concerns about
this gender segregation for reasons connected to the labour market. In the affluent
countries, and beyond, there is a growing need for workers in all caring professions,
including child care, elderly care and the care for individuals with special needs. It will
soon simply be impossible to provide for this growing demand, if recruitment remains
limited to women only (OECD, 2006; Cameron & Moss, 2007). Yet, today, none of
the EU countries had reached the targets that were set for 2006. The Norwegian
government was probably the most successful in the effort to increase the number of
men. Nevertheless the 20% target will not be reached (K. Johanssen, personal
communication, October 9, 2007). At the end of 2006 Norway had 9% of men in
ECE after years of sustained commitment and policy priority, which is the best result
in Europe and probably in the whole world.

Traditionally, it was believed that gender segregation was closely linked with low-
status professions and that, consequently, professionalisation of the child care workforce may facilitate the enrollment of men. However, in countries such as Denmark,
Sweden, New Zealand and in Belgian kindergarten, a high degree of professionalisation
(at bachelors level) coexists with a highly gendered workforce (Cameron, 2006;
Farquhar *et al.*, 2006; Peeters, 2007). As Cameron (2006) and Peeters (2007) note,
professionalisation in terms of extensive training, a unique body of knowledge and a
distinctive occupational identity was achieved with an almost entirely female workforce,
and before efforts were made to recruit more men. In contrast, Scotland has a relatively
low qualified workforce: 40% of the caring professionals do not have Level 2 (Miller,
2008), while the Scottish *Men in Childcare* project succeeded in attracting over 900
men in some form of training for child care (Spence, 2007). Obviously this does not
mean that there is no relationship between professionalisation and gender segregation.

Since its origins in the late nineteenth century, child care has been based on the bour-
geois, patriarchal model of the family, with the male breadwinner and the female carer
as the pillars of both the social and the moral order in society. In different European
countries, carers were traditionally recruited from women of the lower classes and their
profession was based on and legitimated by stereotypical constructions of the ideal

mother (Holmlund, 1999; Vandenbroeck, 2006). Also the women that formed the management of these crèches, or salles d'asile, who were more upper class and intellectual women, entirely conformed to the idealised patriarchal family model (Luc, 1997; Vandenbroeck, 2003). After the World War II, attachment psychology reinforced the gendered caring stereotypes as well as the negative, harmful image of child care, as compared to the ideal mother. But more importantly, attachment psychology also reinforced the construction of the ideal professional as a loving person that was able to facilitate secure attachment with the young child and therefore was modelled after the mother (Singer, 1993; Burman, 1994; Vandenbroeck, 2003). Paradoxically, the feminist movement of the 1970s intensified the image of child care as a female issue (Farquhar *et al.*, 2006). In short, child care has always been considered to be women's work (Cameron *et al.*, 1999; Cameron, 2001). In her study, interviewing recently graduated early childhood educators in New Zealand, Dalli (2002) confirmed that many aspects of the new professionals about their work aligned their professional role with the role of mothers. As Rolfe (2005) claims, these mechanisms tend to reproduce themselves: as the profession is modelled on a mother-like ideal, it attracts merely women, and as the profession is gender segregated, it becomes more difficult for men to enter this workforce.

Men as carers

Simpson (2005) studied men who entered in traditional female jobs. According to his typology, three different types can be observed. 'Seekers' are men who deliberately look for traditional female work; 'finders' initially searched for a more traditional male job, but ended up in a female workforce and 'settlers' are men who have tried different other jobs and, being disappointed, they choose for a traditional female job. The latter can be compared to the 'rethought careers', Cameron *et al.* (1999) describe. It is, however, assumed that the female culture, associated with the profession, may be one of the most important pull-factors that prevent men from joining the caring workforce. In such a female climate, men who enter paid child care work are often thought of as men who are not 'real' men or gay (Farquhar *et al.*, 2006).

This partly explains why, as the experiences in the Scandinavian countries show, actions to employ more men in the provisions for young children are only effective if they step in at all levels, and then over a long period of time. In order to bring more equilibrium into the gender balance, the political will is necessary to make this theme a policy priority for at least 10 years (Moss, 2003). Governmental support for a variety of actions and campaigns is, according to Moss, an important stipulation for success. In their policy documents, the government should continually mention the importance of the presence of men in the provisions for young children. Yet, several programmes and studies have shown that progress can be made by interventions on different levels: the choice process of students, the initial training, as well as the working conditions and job perceptions.

An important role is reserved for the centres that advice on choice of studies and vocational guidance. Men, in particular, who are dissatisfied with their current jobs (rethought career) and had been active in the past in child welfare work, should be alerted to opportunities offered by adult education (Cameron *et al.*, 1999; Peeters, 2007). In addition, action must be taken to better counsel male adolescents in their study choices. In particular, those who are interested in working with children and young people should be brought into contact, via job fairs, with male child care workers who can point out the creative opportunities of a job with children (Rolfe, 2005).

In order to realise a gender-neutral concept of professionalism, the climate in the training courses and the facilities may need to change (Cameron, 2006). The presence of male staff members and the active involvement of fathers in the facilities are essential conditions for achieving a gender-neutral structure of professionalism. Initiatives to attract more male staff members may, therefore, be encouraged but will, in the near future, not produce any spectacular results because qualified male child care workers are simply not available on the labour market (Rolfe, 2005, p. 3). It is, therefore, exceedingly important to develop the initial training courses based on a gender-neutral professionalism and to focus actions on training courses that lead to professions in child care.

The training courses for the child care professions may be integrated in the training institutes where both 'typically male'—generally technical—and 'typically female' professions are taught to avoid isolation of male students (Vandenheede, 2006). Schools must actively recruit male teachers and training supervisors. Male students should preferably be supervised by male supervisors or mentors.

Professionalism in the child care professions should be given a broader interpretation. Countries such as Norway and Denmark, where emphasis is placed on outdoor activities and sports, have been able to construct a different type of professionalism that is gender neutral and were successful in attracting male staff members and fathers (Wohlgemuth, 2003; Hauglund, 2005). A concept of the profession that gives more attention to the social function of child care (Vandenbroeck, 2004), e.g. focus on equal opportunities and community work, also opens up opportunities to attract more men (Meleady & Broadhead, 2002). The experiences of Maori Te Kohanga Reo centres in New Zealand show how the professional cultural climate affects gender-neutral enrollment. Fathers in the Maori Te Kohanga Reo centres are involved and encouraged to volunteer for work in the programmes. This men-friendly climate attracts men to consider becoming a teaching/child care professional in the Maori centres where 30% of the staff is male (Peeters, 2007).

Finally the working conditions also influence the gendered character of the caring work. The offer of predominantly part-time jobs is a pull factor for the employment of men in child care (Peeters, 2005; Rolfe, 2005). In the sectors such as out-of-school care, where there is a great deal of part-time work, one could look for a combination with other jobs so that full-time employment may be realised.

Methods and samples

Unsurprisingly, research on men in child care is rather recent, scarce and involves only very small samples of male carers (Cameron, 2006). Therefore little is known about the students' perspectives on how the gendered culture of the profession is transmitted through overt or covert curricula and how this may affect them. In Flanders, we recently supervised some studies that were carried out in this field with the help of Masters students in Social Work from the Department of Social Welfare Studies at the Gent University in Belgium. In the first two studies (Mannaert, 2006; Vandenheede, 2006), 46 male students were interviewed. Sixteen of them attended adult education for child care and their age varied from 18 to 25 years with one exception: a man of 40 years. In this first group, all of the participants finished secondary school in very different areas of work, including automechanics, paint, agriculture, construction, graphics and trade. Only one of them followed secondary studies in the caring field, but worked in industry for several years before starting his child care studies. Consequently, all adult participants could be considered to have 'rethought careers' (Cameron *et al.*, 1999). Four adult participants did not finish secondary school and four attended one or more years of college, prior to their choice for child care studies, including nursing, management and teaching. None of them finished these bachelor studies.

The other 30 men studied child care in secondary voluntary schools and their age varied between 16 and 20 years. This second group can hardly be considered as having rethought careers, although most of them were one or more years behind in their school career. The topics of the interviews were based on earlier research, including Cameron *et al.* (1999) and Simpson (2005), on earlier experiences in projects for men in child care (for an overview: see Peeters, 2003, 2007), and on literature on pull and push factors and on gender segregation in school (e.g. Dillabough, 2001; Skelton, 2001; Weaver-Hightower, 2003), including both reflections on hegemonic masculinity and aspects of day-to-day teaching practices.

Since many years, authors have highlighted the importance of hidden curricula, including covert and overt gender constructions in textbooks (e.g. Measor & Sikes, 1992; Rifkin, 1998). Although there is an abundance of research on gender construction in textbooks for children (e.g. Evans & Davies, 2000; Gooden & Gooden, 2001) or in subjects such as science (e.g. Elgar, 2004), there is hardly any systematic research of textbooks in child care studies. Moreover, most research is limited to the representations of women in textbooks and does hardly include critical analysis of the representations of men. In our study, representations of men and women were analysed in regard to children, parents and professionals in Flemish textbooks of the secondary voluntary education in child care (Vereecke, 2006). Eight courses were analysed: a sample of 1635 pages, in which 10,487 references to children; 1421 references to parents; 676 references to the care workforce; and 1597 references to other adults (e.g. medical staff) occurred. We will not discuss the latter as this is beyond the scope of this article. Additionally, the textbooks contained 406 visual illustrations (photos and drawings) that were also analysed. As the textbooks use many examples (observations of children or interactions, descriptions of scenes with children at home or in the centres) to illustrate the texts, we attached a special attention to the analysis of these 787 examples. The study combined a quantitative screening, based on Evans and Davies (2000) and Gooden and Gooden (2001), with a qualitative analysis of the context in which the references occurred, based on Elgar (2004).

Results

Choices and reactions

Families are an important source of career advice to young people (Cameron *et al.*, 1999). Most adult respondents confirmed this and said their choice had to a large extent been influenced by friends, a girl friend, their mother or their sister. Yet, only 6 of the 16 adolescent secondary school students can be considered as 'seekers' (Simpson, 2005), meaning that they deliberately chose for the caring sector. The majority were 'finders', boys who rather accidentally ended up in this sector, after negative experiences in other fields and often because others (i.e. educational bureau's) convinced them to make this choice. This does not necessarily imply that 'finders' would not be satisfied with where they end up.

In contrast to the secondary school students, the men in adult education were mostly 'settlers' (Simpson, 2005) or 'rethought careers' (Cameron *et al.*, 1999), meaning that they made a deliberate choice for child care studies, in order to find a job in this field. Most came to this settlement after one or more other choices that did not please them. As one respondent explained:

> I worked during 11 years in agriculture, but this was too lonely a job for me. I prefer to work with people. Later I tried a newspaper shop, and that was a bit better, but not really what I wanted.

In these rethought or settled careers, in 11 of the 16 cases, previous experiences in working with children (baby-sitting or youth work) played a major role in their decision.

The adults claimed to have hardly experienced any negative comments about their choice. Especially men who previously had experience with children (e.g. in youth work), said that their choice was not unexpected for their families. Only three of the men (all without prior experience in youth work) faced initial resistance to their choice by their fathers and in one case also by the mother, although even in these cases the resistance changed into support in a later phase, when their parents became convinced this was a good choice for them. This is similar for the younger students in secondary school. Only very few (three) had negative reactions from their family or close friends. The prevailing feeling was that they felt supported in their choice. The same goes for the reactions of their (almost exclusively feminine) teachers. Neither in adult education, nor in secondary school, did any of the respondents felt discriminated against, although some had the feeling that they were monitored more closely.

This is in contrast with earlier findings in the UK (Cameron *et al.*, 1999). Our findings suggest that the intimate entourage reacted rather positively on their choice, but that especially the younger male students still were afraid of reactions from the larger public and less intimate acquaintances. Often they where reluctant to say what their school study was, in first contacts. As one boy claimed:

> Everybody said this was a good choice for me, since I have a rather social attitude. They support me. It's more the people who don't know me, that react in a strange way. They say it's not a man's job. Therefore it is so important that my family and friends support me.

In the few cases that they were confronted with negative reactions from close peers, they claimed to be able to defend themselves well. As one boy stated:

> In that case, I tell them that I have very good experiences at work, more interesting ones than they may have. I just reply to them: this is what I wish to do.

Consequently, it seems that negative reactions can play an important role, not so much through actually lived reactions from the parents or close friends, but rather through expected reactions of a broader entourage and a general feeling of uneasiness with not being coherent with hegemonic masculinity. One example of this is that some of the boys said they were afraid to be considered gay. It is of course very well possible that our sample was biased, as only men who pursued their child care studies were part of the sample. Consequently, men who dropped out earlier in their studies, or chose other directions, may have been more negatively influenced by their family or peers than those in the sample.

Both the boys in secondary school and the men in adult education argued consistently that it is important for them that there are more public images of men in caring jobs, in order to challenge stereotypical gendered ideas in the broader society. They explicitly asked for male carers in newspapers and magazines, television and movies, as they themselves often knew no men in their field of work.

Internalised constructions about male carers

Most of the adolescent boys in secondary school as well as the men in adult education claimed that their approach to children is 'different' from their female peers. They said men are more strict with the rules, engage more in physical and rough play with the children and make more use of humour. They did not consider this to be problematic but on the contrary they thought very positively about this diversity. They did not claim to be better carers than their female peers, just different, and they attached a value to this diversity. As one participant said:

> A mixed team is better for the child because men and women bring different things, they are each other's complement.

The adolescent boys were all well aware that the presence of a man in a child care centre may cause safety concerns and, however they regretted this suspicion of male carers, they claimed that it did influence their behaviour. As one secondary pupil put it:

> Since the Dutroux-case [a famous case of paedophilia, that was all over the media for a considerable time in Belgium], I was afraid of the reactions of parents and that they would consider me as a paedophile. One must always refrain oneself in physical contacts with children. Like a two year old that can not walk very well and clings on to you. When I cuddled them or gave them a kiss, I always wondered, is it OK to do so? Will people not get wrong ideas about me?

Often the men in adult education did not share this feeling of concern, although one man declared: 'When I will be older, like 40, I will need to find another job, since people will not accept that an older man works with young children. It's a pity, but that's how it is'.

The curriculum

Many of the boys in secondary school complained that some of the subjects were very feminine, including cleaning and ironing, and that some other subjects, such as hygiene, had a very gender-specific content (including for instance care of the nails). They suggested that these subjects would better be optional and that sports and music could be part of the options to choose from. This is for them one of the more important ways of building a more gender-neutral curriculum. Experiences in Scandinavian countries confirm this (Wohlgemuth, 2003; Hauglund, 2005). Additionally most of them were very aware that the textbooks were not neutral. They could give many examples of gender stereotypes in their textbooks as well as in the oral lessons and stated that their textbooks were even more gender stereotyped than in reality. The students said this did not offend them, but they believed it contributed to the general feeling that care is a female work.

One of the most explicit aspect of the hidden curriculum, the boys in secondary school mentioned, is that all of the boys were the only ones in their class, sometimes even in the entire school. They explicitly and consistently deplored this and they also missed 'someone to talk to', not only during courses but also during recess times. In adult education, only five men had a male fellow student in their class. The others were also alone. In contrast with the secondary pupils, the majority of these adults did not seem to miss the presence of other men and felt very comfortable in the group. Only 5 of the 16 did miss the possibility to have other conversations than the usual 'women's talk'.

The work placements are the first real encounters with child care centres for the students and therefore with the profession. The men in our studies were confronted in a very material way with the covert gendered curriculum during their work placements: lack of dressing rooms or toilets for men and staff wearing female uniforms (i.e. an apron). As Evans (2002) also found with regard to nurses, the uniform, because it projects a feminine image, may have a negative influence on the acceptance of men. In contrast to this explicit message about the workplace, the men felt very welcomed by their female colleagues and consistently stated that they have never been overtly discriminated against. The majority of them were convinced that when they would apply for a job, after having finished their studies, they would easily be employed. However, many of them cited examples of being treated differently. One man spoke about his coffee being served, while the female colleagues had to serve themselves, but more importantly, several men said they had been assigned different and stereotypical tasks compared to their female colleagues, such as outdoor play, construction play and creative activities. This was experienced by the respondents as receiving less responsibilities, 'being a visitor rather than a colleague'. As one man declared:

> When a child needed a change, the [female] child care worker said 'let me do that'. The women often asked me 'Are you doing OK?', even with the most simple tasks, everyone could do. In fact I was there for the amusement of the children, not for the care. When a toddler needed some help and I wanted to assist him, they said to me: 'You can go to the playground with the others, I will do that'. I don't think they did this on purpose, it's rather unconscious.

Cameron *et al.* (1999) found that men in child care were not always trusted by the parents. This is not confirmed in our studies. On the contrary, the men in adult education had very positive reactions from parents who were happy that a man joined the team. Eight of the 16 adult men reported examples of fathers having more contacts and exchanges with them than with their female colleagues.

The textbooks

The quantitative and qualitative analyses of the textbooks show the existence of a consistent sexist hidden curriculum.

Children were almost always portrayed as neutral (it) or male (him). The percentage of children portrayed as girls (her), varied from 0.9% to 1.2%. This was the case, both for plain texts and for examples of observations of children in the textbooks, with the exception of textbooks that were only about care: there, girls were more present in the examples. In the illustrations, children were most often depicted as sexless and 'neutral'. When their sex was obvious (mostly in photographs, seldom in drawings), again, the vast majority of the children depicted, were boys. A closer look at the context in which the children were depicted, revealed an even more sexist approach. When the text was about aggression in children, for instance, the children that showed aggression in the example were always boys. When children were playing, they performed very gender-stereotypical play: boys played with cars, balls, blocks and other construction materials, while girls consistently played with dolls. Only in two examples, on a total of 787, children performed a play activity that was not stereotypical.

As far as the parents were concerned, they were referred to in neutral terms (i.e. the plural form parents) or as mothers. The percentage of explicit references to fathers varied from 3.7% to 10.2%. The highest percentage was in courses on education. In courses on care, fathers were virtually absent. In the illustrations, only 12 men occurred in the 1635 pages (less than 1%). The content analyses revealed that all care activities were performed by mothers. The textbooks stated that fathers do play a role, but examples of this role were not given. When fathers performed in examples, it was most often in a negative role (e.g. a father does not hear the baby crying in the night or a father scolds the child). All household activities (cleaning, washing, cooking, etc.) were done by mothers, while the fathers did the gardening and went to their offices.

The references to staff were almost entirely references to female staff. References to male workers never exceeded 0.9%. In the 1635 pages of text that were analysed, not one male carer occurred in an example, except in the context of school age child care and more specifically in outdoor play (such as building huts). There were very few illustrations of staff, all of them women. The management in the textbooks was also 100% female.

Discussion

Child care has always been and continues to be a female profession. There is a growing consensus among policy makers, academia and the field that this is problematic for economic reasons (shortages on the labour market), for educational reasons (broadening the repertoires of the possible) and for social reasons (equal opportunities for men and women). As Cameron and Moss (2007) state, there are urgent reasons to move the professionalisation beyond the old mother-like, low status profession.

> This means recognising the gendered assumptions that have underpinned so much care work until now, and the way these assumptions have served to sustain gender inequality and poor quality employment. (Cameron & Moss, 2007, p. 156)

However, things have not significantly changed over the last few decades, and very few men enter the caring workforce. Recent studies in Flanders and internationally reveal some of the factors that, together, make out the *habitus* (Bourdieu & Wacquant, 1996) that inhibit change in this field, but they also show some ways forward, including a multi-level approach that intervened on multiple aspects of the training of the workforce.

In the case of Flanders, the curriculum reinforces the mother-like gendered construction of the workforce by linking courses on care and education to household and hygienic activities that are considered by male students to be inappropriate. There is an urgent need to revisit the curriculum and introduce variation, including sports and music. Danish examples, introducing sports, have shown that this may significantly influence the attendance by male students (Wohlgemuth, 2003). There is also a need to incorporate child care studies with other, more 'traditionally male' studies in one school, in order to enable male students to socialise with male peers during recess times, especially when adolescents are concerned.

In addition, the Flemish textbooks support a very stereotypical and sexist construction of care work, with regards to children, parents and staff. It is urgent to organise systematic screenings of textbooks in order to clean them from the most blatant stereotypes. Training of trainers on gender awareness in child care and early childhood education may be most welcome, as the stereotypes not only persist in the textbooks, but also in the oral comments during the courses.

The male students in our Flemish sample did not encounter much public disagreement, or disapprovement by parents, unlike their UK peers. On the contrary they feel supported by their family and close friends and they feel welcomed by female colleagues and parents, but not always for reasons that the men themselves would cherish. Indeed, in the workplace, men are often very well aware that they are 'the exception' as they do not have separate changing rooms or toilets. They are confronted with stereotypical thinking and tokenism, as they feel they have to perform, according to gendered roles where care is not for them, while outdoor play is. They have also interiorised some gendered constructions of the work and feel that they may be distrusted in the presence of children. Their narratives show that gendered opinions also affect the women in the workforce and in order to make the care work more gender neutral, actions towards both men and women are needed.

Men who choose for child care, can be very lonely, being the only boy in the class or even in the entire school. They miss 'pals' to talk to about other things than 'women's talk' and to share their sense of humour. Many of the men we interviewed, explicitly asked for the possibility of male networks, where they can exchange these experiences. During the research process, we set up an Internet chat room that was used by the secondary school students for this purpose.

In England and Scotland men-only child care orientation programmes are very successful. The *Men in Childcare* project (Edinburgh) has run induction and taster courses, and access courses for more advanced training. The *Men in Childcare* project had 900 men who followed some form of training after a men-only introduction course. In Edinburgh, there are now 25 fully qualified men working in child care settings. Another 70 men are currently in training and 40 of them will be fully qualified in June 2007 (Spence, 2007).

We unveiled some aspects of a curriculum that is embedded in what we would call an overt and covert hegemonic feminity of the profession. This seems to affect younger secondary school students who are still 'seeking' a suitable job for them and who are in their adolescence more, than it affects adult 'settlers', who come to the child care workforce after negative experiences in other fields, but having good experiences in youth work. Both groups, however, would welcome more general campaigns that challenge stereotypical male and female job descriptions. National campaigns to attract more men have been successful in Denmark, Norway, the UK and Belgium. A campaign, launched by VBJK and the governmental agency for child care in Flanders in 2003, showed that media campaigns can have significant effects. The campaign increased the number of men working in child care in the Flemish part of Belgium considerably. In 2002, before the campaign was set up, only 0.9% of the workforce was male. In 2005 the number of men increased to 2.08%, and in 2006 2.3% of the workforce in child care was men. In absolute figures, this is an increase from 142 men in 2002 to 415 men in 2006 (Kind en Gezin, 2007). We can conclude from this campaign that it is possible to attract more men in the caring workforce, especially adults with a rethought career, but also that the effects of such a campaign are limited in time. Persistent, long-term strategies are needed. If we additionally wish to also influence the school choice of younger male adolescents, multiple actions over longer periods of time are necessary, combining revisions of the curricula and textbooks, training of trainers, creating networking possibilities for men and sustained media campaigns that offer positive role models for men in caring work. The campaigns should not merely aim to reach men or boys, but also women in the care workforce, teachers in early childhood education, school advisory offices and labour offices.

References

Bourdieu, P. & Wacquant, L. (1996) *An invitation to reflexive sociology* (Cambridge, MA, Polity Press).

Burman, E. (1994) *Deconstructing developmental psychology* (London, Routledge).

Cameron, C. (2001) Promise or problem? A review on the literature on men working in early childhood services, *Gender, Work and Organisation*, 8(4), 430–453.

Cameron, C. (2006) Male workers and professionalism, *Contemporary Issues in Early Childhood*, 7(1), 68–79.

Cameron, C. & Moss, P. (2007) *Care work in Europe: current understandings and future directions* (London, Routledge).

Cameron, C., Moss, P. & Owen, S. (1999) *Men in the nursery: gender and caring work* (London, Paul Chapman).

Council of Ministers of the European Union (1992, 21 January) *Recommendations on childcare* (10258/91) (Brussels, EU).

Dalli, C. (2002) Being a early childhood teacher: images of professional practice and professional identity during the experience of starting childcare, *New Zealand Journal of Educational Studies*, 37(1), 73–85.

Dillabough, J. A. (2001) Gender theory and research in education: modernist traditions and emerging contemporary themes, in: B. Francis & C. Skelton (Eds) *Investigating gender: contemporary perspectives in education* (Buckingham/Philadelphia, PA, Open University), 11–26.

Elgar, A. G. (2004) Science textbooks for lower secondary schools in Brunei: issues of gender equity, *International Journal of Science Education*, 26(7), 875–894.

European Commission Childcare Network (1993, 21–22 May) *Men as carers: report of an international seminar* (Ravenna, EC Childcare Network).

Evans, J. A. (2002) Cautious caregivers: gender stereotypes and the sexualisation of men nurses' touch, *Journal of Advanced Nursing*, 40(4), 441–448.

Evans, L. & Davies, K. (2000) No sissy boys here: a content analysis of the representation of masculinity in elementary school reading textbooks, *Sex Roles*, 42(3/4), 255–270.

Farquhar, S., Cablk, L., Buckingham, A., Butler, D. & Ballantyne, R. (2006) *Men at work: sexism in early childhood education* (Porirua, Childforum Research Network).

Gooden, A. M. & Gooden, M. A. (2001) Gender representation in notable children's picture books: 1995–1999, *Sex Roles*, 45(1/2), 89–101.

Hauglund, E. (2005) Men in childcare in Norway, paper presented at the *Men in Childcare Conference*, National Children's Bureau, London, 20 September.

Holmlund, K. (1999) Child-cribs for the poor and kindergartens for the rich: two directions for early childhood institutions in Sweden (1854–1930), *History of Education*, 28(2), 143–155.

Jensen, J. (1998) Men as worker in childcare services, in: C. Owen, C. Cameron & P. Moss (Eds) *Men as workers in services for young children: issues of gender workforce* (London, Institute of Education), 118–136.

Kind en Gezin (2007) *Internal report. Aantal mannen in de kinderopvang* [Internal report. Number of men in child care] (Brussels, Author).

Lamb, M. E. (1975) Fathers: forgotten contributors to child development, *Human Development*, 18(4), 245–266.

Luc, J. (1997) *L'invention du jeune enfant au XIXème siècle. De la salle d'asile à l'école maternelle* [The invention of the young child in the 19th century. From the 'salle d'asile' toward the 'école maternelle'] (Paris, Belin).

Mannaert, N. (2006) *Mannen in een gendergesegregeerde opleiding* (Onuitgegeven Meesterproef) (Gent, Vakgroep Sociale Agogiek, Ugent).

Measor, L. & Sikes, P. (1992) *Introduction to education: gender and schools* (London, Briddles).

Meleady, C. & Broadhead, P. (2002) Diversity: the norm, not the exception, *Children in Europe*, 2(2), 11–15.

Miller, L. (2008) Developing new professional roles in the early years, in: L. Miller & C. Cable (Eds) *Professionalism in the early years* (London, Hodder Arnold), 20–31.

Moss, P. (Ed) (1995) *Quality targets in services for young children* (Brussels, European Commission).

Moss, P. (1996) *A review of services for young children in the EU 1990–1995* (Brussels, European Commission Network on Childcare and Other Measures to Reconcile Employment and Family Responsibilities).

Moss, P. (2003) Wie is de begeleider in de kinderopvang? Kinderen in Europa [Who is the early childhood professional? Children in Europe], *KIDDO*, 4(7), 11–15.

OECD. (2006) *Starting strong II: early childhood education and care* (Paris, Author).

Peeters, J. (2003) Men in childcare: an action-research in Flanders, *International Journal for Equity and Innovation in Early Childhood,* 1(1), 72–83.

Peeters, J. (2005) Promoting diversity and equality in early childhood care and education. Men in childcare, in: H. Schonfeld, S. O'Brien & T. Walsh (Eds) *Questions of Quality* (Dublin, CEDCE), 152–162.

Peeters, J. (2007) Including men in early childhood education: insights from the European perspective, *New Zealand Research in Early Childhood Education,* 10, 15–24.

Rifkin, B. (1998) Gender representation in foreign language textbooks: a case study of textbooks in Russian, *Modern Language Journal,* 82(2), 217–236.

Rolfe, H. (2005) *Men in childcare* (Working paper series no. 35) (London, Equal Opportunities Commission).

Simpson, R. (2005) Men in non-traditional occupations: career entry, career orientation and experience of role strain, *Gender, Work and Organisation,* 12, 363–380.

Singer, E. (1993) Shared care for children, *Theory & Psychology,* 3(4), 429–449.

Skelton, C. (2001) Typical boys? Theorizing masculinity in educational settings, in: B. Francis & C. Skelton (Eds) *Investigating gender: contemporary perspectives in education* (Buckingham/Philadelphia, PA, Open University), 164–176.

Spence, K. (2007) Men in childcare, Paper presented at the *International 'Men in Childcare' Seminar,* ESSSE, Lyon, 27 April.

Vandenbroeck, M. (2003) From crèches to childcare: constructions of motherhood and inclusion/exclusion in the history of Belgian infant care, *Contemporary Issues in Early Childhood,* 4(2), 137–148.

Vandenbroeck, M. (2004) *In verzekerde bewaring. Honderd vijftig jaar kinderen, ouders en kinderopvang* [Hundred fifty years of children, parents and child care] (Amsterdam, SWP).

Vandenbroeck, M. (2006) The persistent gap between education and care: a 'history of the present' research on Belgian child care provision and policy, *Paedagogica Historica,* 42(3), 363–383.

Vandenheede, E. (2006) *Gendersegregatie in het onderwijs: jongens in de opleiding kinderzorg* [Gender segregation in education: boys in early childhood education] (Onuitgegeven Meesterproef) (Unpublished Masters' Thesis) (Gent, Vakgroep Sociale Agogiek, Ugent).

Vereecke, K. (2006) *De opleiding kinderzorg in genderperspectief: een onderzoek naar het lesmateriaal* [The training for child care from a gender perspective: a research into the training materials] (Onuitgegeven Meesterproef) Unpublished Masters' thesis (Gent, Vakgroep Sociale Agogiek, Ugent).

Weaver-Hightower, M. (2003) The 'boy turn' in research on gender and education, *Review of Educational Research,* 73(4), 471–498.

Wohlgemuth, U. G. (2003) Meer mannelijke opvoeders [More male educators], *KIDDO,* 7, 30–31.

Entrances and exits: changing perceptions of primary teaching as a career for men

Mary Thornton and Patricia Bricheno
University of Hertfordshire, UK

Introduction

The number of men in teaching has always been small, particularly in early childhood, and a variety of reasons have been put forward as to why this is the case. At a general level, in most societies, work is gendered, there is a continuing sexual division of labour (Cockburn, 1991), and teaching, especially in the early years, is a predominantly female occupation. More specifically, Mills suggests so few men teach because of

> ... poor wages in relation to the work performed; limited career path for those not seeking administrative roles; the labelling of male primary school teachers as homosexual or not 'real men'; the current media spotlight on allegations of child abuse; the fear of being labelled a paedophile. (2005, p. 5)

Hegemonic masculinity serves to restrict the career options available to men (Mac an Ghaill, 1994). To go against this expectation requires men contemplating teaching as a career to be particularly confident about their sexuality and their ability to counter imputations of paedophilic intentions.

In the 1990s, there was considerable suspicion of men in teaching, particularly in the primary sector; concerns were expressed about whether men should be encouraged into early years work (Pringle, 1998), and questions were raised about the sexuality of men who worked in primary teaching (Thornton, 2001). This linked to public concerns about child protection issues (Whitehead, 2002); Howson (cited in Haughton, 2002) suggested that the increased focus on child protection following the Children Act 1989 may have impacted negatively on the recruitment of male primary school teachers. However, such concerns may now have lessened, in part because of the implementation of mandatory police checks on everyone who works with children.

So, there have been some significant disincentives to men becoming teachers of young children. However, there have also been incentives. Once in teaching men have a marked tendency to move swiftly up the career ladder, disproportionately occupying higher paid and higher status positions (Drudy *et al.*, 2005; Thornton & Bricheno, 2006). This represents a clear benefit to those men who choose to make counter-stereotypical career choices, such as teaching.

Our research has found that the kinds of concerns outlined by Mills (2005) were shared by many new male entrants to teaching in 1998, but that they were not prevalent among the reasons given by men who had left or intended to leave teaching in 2005. This could suggest that initial concerns about becoming a teacher are either mistaken, or overcome, during the course of teachers careers, or that there have been changes in wider society that make such concerns less important than they once were.

Concerns about becoming a teacher in 1998

In 1998, in collaboration with Professor Ivan Reid, then at the University of Loughborough, we undertook a large-scale survey, partly funded by the TTA, into 'Students' Reasons for Choosing Primary Teaching as a Career' (Reid & Thornton, 2000). This research involved a questionnaire survey of, and follow-up interviews with, new (1998 entry) primary teaching students drawn from 14 different Higher Education institutions in England. The sample comprised 1611 questionnaire responses and 143 follow-up interviews (of which 2 were not identified by gender). First-year undergraduates and PGCE primary students across four chartered and seven non-chartered universities plus three university colleges were included in this survey. The institutional sample was broadly representative of Higher Education ITE providers and the gender sample was close to then current intake figures of approximately 15% male, 85% female. Similar studies have since been carried out by Carrington (2002), Drudy *et al.* (2005), Hobson *et al.* (2005) and Hargreaves *et al.* (2007).

All of these studies concluded that both male and female student teachers chose to teach for positive reasons, e.g. they enjoyed working with children, believed it would bring high job satisfaction and would be a challenging but rewarding career.

However, within that context, we found that men were more likely than women to be attracted to primary teaching by the conditions of service (such as long holidays, index-linked pension and career prospects), while women were more likely than men to be attracted to teaching because it involved work with children, fitted well with parenthood, and because they wanted to make a difference (Thornton & Bricheno, 2006).

Our student interviewees were volunteers who self-identified in the survey. Clearly, these students were a self-selected group from the much larger survey sample. However, it is still a large sample and their perceptions and their concerns about becoming teachers are illuminating.

Three questions in particular elicited the concerns and reservations shown in Table 1:

(1) What do you think might put people off becoming primary teachers?
(2) What do you think should and could be done to encourage more people to enter primary teaching?
(3) Do you have any reservations about primary teaching as your career?

The main concerns expressed by both men and women about entering the teaching profession centred on pay, workload and the status of teachers. Concerns were expressed about teacher's pay levels and their perceived inappropriateness for graduate entrants to teaching, for attracting the more able/highly qualified into teaching and for 'breadwinners'.

> Pay is basically the BIG issue and responsibility and paperwork. I wasn't aware how much they have to do. Seen as a women's profession and therefore people do not want to go into it and it is not seen as a reputable profession. (Female PGCE)

> Pay being linked to pupil performance. (Male PGCE)

Lack of teacher autonomy and the somewhat heartfelt cry of 'let teachers teach' are echoed in many sections of the interview data, where respondents emphasised the burdensome nature of non-teaching duties, be they administrative, paper-based or out-of-class activities.

> Paper work increasing—new strategies every year, with a new curriculum next year which will more than likely change or be revised, followed by more changes in practice with a new emphasis ... you get the point. (Male PGCE)

> ... the workload, it's not 9 to 3 pm, it's more like 8 to 8 pm. (Male BA-QTS)

> Workload is horrendous. (Female PGCE)

> Being tired all the time and working almost non-stop for the same money as I was getting as a secretary. (Female UG)

> Funding of proper administration in schools—let teachers teach. (Male PGCE)

These successfully recruited trainees also had concerns about the 'bad press' that teaching had attracted and the apparent low status of teachers.

Table 1.   Primary ITE students' concerns about being a teacher in 1998, by gender

	1998	
Issue	Male (%) (*n* = 20)	Female (%) (*n* = 121)
Pay	70.0	68.6
Status	65.0	47.1
Workload	50.0	63.6
Government initiatives	35.0	43.0
Gender issues	30.0	5.0
Behaviour	25.0	14.9
Stress/health	10.0	16.5
Performance pay	5.0	4.1
Management	5.0	0.0

Teachers ... are the first in the firing line when 'standards' are not acceptable but the last to be praised. (Male PGCE)

I think that better opinion from the government and the public of teaching is required. I think that teachers should stop getting the blame for society's ills. (Female PGCE)

The teaching profession needs to have a higher status in the eyes of the public—too often it is seen as a job that people do because they can't think of anything else to do. (Female PGCE)

Still seen as a ladies' job, should be more of a profession like secondary teaching. You are a professional but people do not see you as one. (Female PGCE)

However, although important to both men and women, teacher status was more often referred to by men and workload more often referred to by women.

Low public esteem. From a male perspective, pay, as a first income, this is not good and prospects are not good either. You reach the ceiling and are stuck. Teaching is seen as a female profession, particularly the early years. KS1 for me was difficult as the younger ones need more 'mothering'. Primary teaching is seen as an odd profession for a man to be in. (Male PGCE)

Teachers are not seen as professionals. They are not portrayed positively in the media— everyone remembers bad teachers. We need a more professional profile. Teachers have the stigma of being left-wing softie profession. The NUT is a militant/political body, represented as trade union. We need our own professional body. There is the impression that primary teachers do a 9–3.30 job and anyone can do this, this is ignorance on the part of the media and others. (Male PGCE)

The amount of paperwork! I honestly never realised there was so much. I have spoken to teachers about it, they themselves have commented on the fact that it has become a lot worse over the years! (Female BA-QTS)

I won't be doing it for the rest of my life [I used to think I would], because of the amount of work and lack of reward. (Female PGCE)

Like other researchers in the field (Johnston *et al.*, 1999; Smedley, 1999), we found that issues relating to the gender of the teacher were of far greater concern for men in 1998, at the start of their training, than they were for women, and that men more frequently expressed concerns about pupil behaviour than did women.

> People's opinion of males, questioning men's intentions, surprised me! (Male UG)

> There is a stigma attached. In the 1970s in my primary school, I had male teachers. They have gone because it is a cultural thing. Primary teaching is seen as a 'sissy job', as effeminate. It does not have a macho profile, the pay is not good and it is not a high achieving or competitive career. (Male PGCE)

On the other hand, more women than men referred to the number of government initiatives and had concerns about their future stress levels.

> The new pay proposals will bring a change in the working environment and bring unpleasantness. In primary teaching the ethos is team working, so that the staff bond together and these proposals threaten that. (Female PGCE)

> Worried about stress levels and how much life outside school will be affected. (Female BA-QTS)

> Yes, the pressure, what is expected of you. All the teachers I have met seem to have so much to do. This worries me. I want to have a life as well. (Female PGCE)

It is interesting that pay was cited as one of the major disincentives to teaching in 1998. Significant increases in pay and changes to the pay structure for teachers were proposed around this time but had yet to materialise in pay packets.

In 1998, there were also some clear signs of government attempting to accentuate the positive aspects of teaching and to attract positive publicity for teachers. The Green Paper (DfEE, 1998b) 'Meeting the childcare challenge: a framework and consultation document', had just been published. It set out a new deal for teachers in the form of a new pay and career structure, and more formalised professional development, with the stated purposes of:

- improving quality through workplace reform,
- imposing professional standards on newly qualified teachers,
- enhancing career prospects through clarifying routes to promotion and higher pay scales,
- introducing numeracy and literacy strategise in primary schools,
- setting up a General Teaching Council (GTC), and
- turning teaching into 'a first class profession'.

It was this document that introduced the idea of performance-related pay for teachers, with movement to a new, improved salary scale dependent on pupil achievements. However, the Green Paper was not well received by teachers at the time. They felt it would be divisive, introduce competitiveness into a collegial working environment and would not be properly funded (Bricheno & Thornton, 1999). It also introduced more controls over teachers, their training and the curriculum they taught. Feelings among those successfully recruited during 1998 were of teaching being a low-status profession, one that was under paid and overworked, and often criticised in the media. There was clearly still much to be done.

Research undertaken in 2005 explored teachers reasons for leaving teaching and it is against this later data that we can explore whether or not the perceptions and concerns of leaving teachers in any way 'mirror' the concerns expressed by new entrants back in 1998.

Reasons for leaving teaching in 2005

In 2005, we placed advertisements in newspapers and magazines, inviting teachers who had already left, or were about to leave the profession, to complete an online survey about their reasons for leaving. The questionnaire enabled respondents to write as much as desired in answer to questions about reasons for leaving teaching and planned or envisaged post-teaching work destinations. Three hundred and seventy-one teachers and ex-teachers responded, across all age phases of education. We found that in general they gave many similar reasons to those reported elsewhere, for example: high workload, poor pay, and low status and morale (Spear *et al.*, 2000); workload, government initiatives, stress, pupil behaviour, pay and school management/leadership (Barmby & Coe, 2004). Workload and pay feature in both Spear *et al.* and Barmby and Coe's work, but it is interesting to note the presence of new factors in the 2004 work. Although stress has been a recurring issue in teacher retention (Sturman, 2002; Smithers & Robinson, 2004), school management and pupil behaviour appear to be relatively new concerns. We found, in common with other studies, that pupil behaviour was frequently mentioned as a reason for leaving in 2005 (but of relatively minor concern to our new entrants in 1998).

Our 2005 leavers from the Primary sector gave government initiatives as the most common reason (46.2%) for leaving teaching, while 25% cited pupil behaviour. Pay (12.5%) and status (10.3%) were mentioned far less often than in 1998, and issues relating to the gender of the teacher barely featured at all. Bullying by more senior staff emerged as a reason for leaving although was not mentioned as a possible worry by new entrants in 1998. Do these differences indicate that the pressures of teaching have changed in recent years?

For this group of teachers, government initiatives, workload and pupil behaviour seemed more pressing reasons for leaving than pay or the image/status of teaching (the major concerns of our new entrants in 1998). These differences may be explained by the unusual nature of the methodology and sample of leaving teachers, consisting of a self-selecting group of teachers who felt strongly enough to respond to national advertisements and complete an online survey, but they may also indicate that the nature of teachers work has changed and that the concerns that teachers express about teaching in 2005 are somewhat different to those that were prevalent in 1998.

Focussing on men and women teaching in the Primary sector, we found some interesting gender differences (see Table 2). Men seemed to be more concerned

Table 2.   Primary teachers' reasons for leaving teaching in 2005, by gender

Issue	2005	
	Male (%) (*n* = 34)	Female (%) (*n* = 150)
Government initiatives	57.6	44.0
Behaviour	35.3	22.7
Workload	26.5	30.7
Pay	20.6	10.7
Performance pay	17.6	11.3
Poor management	8.8	13.3
Stress/health	5.9	15.3
Status	5.9	11.3
Bullying	5.9	7.3

about government initiatives, and, as in 1998, about pupil behaviour, pay and performance-related pay. Women, on the other hand, expressed more concern about stress/health and, in contrast to 1998, the status of teachers.

Workload, poor management and bullying were mentioned by similar proportions of both men and women, suggesting no particular gender difference.

[I was] dealing with extremely disruptive pupils, so that I would be actually teaching for less than 50% of actual teaching hours. I was working every evening during the week and at least one day per weekend, whereas my friends in alternative jobs had much more free time out of normal working hours. At the time, the pay was not as good as it is now, but I found the working hours intolerable. (Male Primary)

Targets, unrealistic demands by people in government who have never taught. (Male Primary)

Pay is uncompetitive with peers in private sector with less responsibility and much shorter hours. (Male Primary)

Teachers have too few rights and are expected to do far too much. We don't have the respect of the children or of their parents and this is made worse by the way the government treats us ... We are not treated as professionals—everything is too prescribed. The pay isn't bad, but what we're expected to do for it is just impossible if we're to have any kind of life. We are respected by no one. (Female Primary)

Until the status of teachers and the wider school function is restored, there will be a spiral of poor morale (staff and pupils), bad behaviour, desperate government measures and declining educational achievement. I'm glad I had the option to leave—many don't. (Female Primary)

The insidious undermining of self-esteem through lack of full confidence and trust by the government, parents, the public. The lack of appreciation of the responsibility, knowledge and skills and physical stamina required to teach. The crassly mistaken ideas of policy-makers. (Female Primary)

Similarities and differences: 1998 entrances, 2005 exits

In Table 3, we can see that the concerns of new entrants in 1998 and those of leavers in 2005 are different. This could be explained by the longer experience and greater immersion into the culture of teaching of leavers; by changes in individual life contexts (marriage, children) or changes in priorities and expectations (related to teachers themselves as individuals and groups); or it might be explained by wider changes in society and the socio-economic and cultural context in which teachers work takes place (and, of course, by an interaction between all these things).

Although we cannot talk about percentage decreases and increases for these two quite different samples, it is illuminating to focus on the changes in emphasis that are indicated in Table 3. In 2005, reservations about teaching shifted towards an increase in concern about performance pay, management, bullying and pupil behaviour and towards a decrease in concern about workload, status and pay in general. Only concerns about Government initiatives and stress/health seem to be relatively unchanged.

The leavers sample may be unusual, but our findings regarding a general decrease in the citation of pay as an area of concern are supported by the House of Commons Education and Skills Committee (2004). They reported that pay was no longer considered the main issue in terms of teacher retention, while Hargreaves *et al.*'s (2007) research found that teachers' pay was now much less likely to be seen as an area of concern, rather pay was seen increasingly as a positive feature of a teaching career. This reflects changes to teacher's salaries and pay structures that have taken place since the 1998 Green Paper, and which appear to have had a positive impact on perceptions of pay in the intervening period. Pay is certainly less of an issue for leavers in 2005 than it was for entrants in 1998, as can been seen in Table 4. However, while in 1998 it was of major concern to both men and women entrants, in 2005 a gender difference emerged, with pay of greater concern to men than women.

Pupils' behaviour was a concern for men entering primary teaching in 1998 and is one of the most prominent reasons for men leaving the profession in 2005. On the

Table 3. Comparison of recruits (1998) and leavers (2005) concerns

Issue	1998 (%) (n = 141)	2005 (%) (n = 184)	Concerns in 2005 seem to be:
Workload	61.7	29.9	Less relevant
Pay	68.8	12.5	Less relevant
Status	49.6	10.3	Less relevant
Gender issues	8.5	Not raised	Less relevant
Behaviour	16.3	25.0	More relevant
Performance pay	4.3	12.5	More relevant
Management	0.7	12.5	More relevant
Bullying	Not raised	7.1	More relevant
Government initiatives	41.8	46.2	Relatively unchanged
Stress/health	15.6	13.6	Relatively unchanged

Table 4. Differences in concerns between entrants (1998) and leavers (2005), by gender

Issue	1998 Male entrants (%) (n = 20)	2005 Male leavers (%) (n = 34)	1998 Female entrants (%) (n = 121)	2005 Female leavers (%) (n = 150)
Government initiatives	35.0	57.6	43.0	44.0
Behaviour	25.0	35.3	14.9	22.7
Workload	50.0	26.5	63.6	30.7
Pay	70.0	20.6	68.6	10.7
Performance pay	5.0	17.6	4.1	11.3
Management	5.0	8.8	0	13.3
Status	65.0	5.9	47.1	11.3
Stress/health	10.0	5.9	16.5	15.3
Bullying	Not raised	5.9	Not raised	7.3
Gender issues	30.0	Not raised	5.0	Not raised

other hand, if we look at male and female attitudes to teaching children, we notice that in 1998 the main reason among both male and female students for entering the profession was the enjoyment of working with children. In 2005, very few of those leaving teaching mentioned this. Five men (14.7%) made positive comments; two talked about wanting to give children more fun, two talked about the government initiatives that got in the way of children's education but only one (2.9%) talked positively about children, saying 'Pupils are great'. In contrast, 35 women (23.3%) expressed their enjoyment in teaching children, their love of children and their love of the job and their sadness at their need to leave the profession:

> Yes, they are taking out the enjoyment of teaching and changing the reasons I started and trained to be a teacher. (Female Primary)

> I have been a teacher and Senco for over 20 years in the same school. The pressure is now so great with the continual drive to address new initiatives that I am only now really teaching for the money. All the fun and real enjoyment has largely disappeared. (Female Primary)

> I love teaching and it has been a difficult decision, but I will be leaving next year when my son goes to secondary (I will have been teaching for only three years). I know an awful lot of teachers feel as I do. The children are not the problem and neither is the actual teaching—it's all the other unnecessary rubbish that goes with it. (Female Primary)

Whatever the reason or explanation, men's stated concerns about teaching appear different in 2005 from those expressed in 1998. Male leavers in 2005 were less concerned about workload, pay, status, gender issues and work-related stress than 1998 entrants, but more concerned about government initiatives and children's behaviour. Women leavers in 2005 similarly expressed less concern than did 1998 entrants about workload, status and pay, but had similar levels of concern about work-related stress and government initiatives.

There are some clear differences between the perceptions of men and women as entrants in 1998 and as leavers in 2005. In 1998, both men and women were concerned about pay levels. This was not a predominant concern among leavers, but it was mentioned by twice as many men than women. While pay scales have undoubtedly improved since 1998, men can still earn more money outside of teaching (Dalton & Chung, 2004). Note also that the issue of performance pay, introduced following the 1998 Green Paper, was more prominent among reasons for leaving in 2005 than it was an area of concern for new entrants in 1998; and that this was particularly so for men.

Discussion

Has anything happened in wider society that may have prompted these different responses? In 1998, our new entrants talked about the 'bad press' teachers received.

> It certainly doesn't help that the teachers have such a bad deal in the press. You know, every time you open a newspaper you hardly hear anything good being said about the teachers, it's always like, 'Oh the teachers are on strike again', and the teachers are, you know, do this and they get a very bad press report ... I think their status is low ... I think rather than the government always saying teachers must do this, must do that and have to prove themselves and so on, they should occasionally praise them and say yes they are doing a good job. (Reid & Thornton, 2000, p. 46)

More recently, the DfES Teacher Status Project (Hargreaves *et al.*, 2007) has found that news coverage of teachers and teaching changed significantly between the early 1990s and 2005, and that it has become increasingly positive and supportive of them.

> While much coverage focused on confrontation between teacher unions and government or government-related institutions, there was markedly less emphasis on confrontation—and concomitantly more emphasis on support and help to teachers—in the most recent period ... Earlier news coverage of the 'teacher bashing' mould has given way to a more supportive and less confrontational style of reporting, which gives teachers a prominent 'voice' and recognises, as genuine, the problems and pressures faced by teachers. (Hargreaves *et al.*, 2007, pp. 25–26)

This recent work on the status of teachers (Hargreaves *et al.*, 2007) provides substantial evidence that the representation of teachers in the media is now significantly more positive than it was 10 years ago and that this may in part be due to wider political and social changes.

Prime Minister Blair's constant refrain of 'Education, Education, Education', from his election in 1997, and the conscientious efforts of his ministers to reshape and improve the image of teachers and teaching within the minds and hearts of the British public may well have begun the move towards more positive stories being told about teachers within the media, and may have helped to enhanced public perceptions about teachers and teaching.

The previous Conservative Government had imposed significant changes on teachers, such as the National Curriculum (DES, 1989), national tests, OFSTED inspections, league tables, training days and new contracts, while at the same time battling against teacher strikes over pay and conditions, and engaging in what might be called the 'teacher bashing' cited above. The '3 Wise Men Report' (Alexander *et al.*, 1992), produced in one month and much discussed in the public domain, argued that standards were falling, primary teaching was stuck in the Plowden philosophy of progressive child-centred education, that there should be more streaming, more whole class teaching of separate subjects by subject specialists, and that primary teachers lacked the necessary subject expertise to teach the National Curriculum. Just one year later, John Patten (then Conservative Secretary of State for Education) proposed a 'Mum's Army' (TES, 18 June 1993) of non-graduate and differently trained nursery and KS1 teachers. Both the '3 Wise Men Report' and Patten's proposal were highly controversial and may have served to undermine confidence in primary teachers in the eyes of the general public, and to lower perceptions of the status of the profession.

In comparison to their immediate Conservative predecessors, successive Labour Secretaries of State for Education have spoken more about teacher professionalism and trust rather than criticising teachers and blaming them for poor standards in education. Estelle Morris, as the newly appointed Secretary of State for Education in 2001, said:

> This pamphlet ... is about the next steps we must take to raise standards in our schools yet higher. It focuses on those at the heart of raising standards: the talented and dedicated professionals who staff our schools and teach our children. And it signals a new era of trust in our professionals on the part of Government. (2001, p. 1)

She went on to say:

> Our teachers and school staff are a national asset of priceless value. But as a nation we have not always treated them as such. In the last four years we have begun to put that right. Investment is at record levels, teacher numbers are up and so is pay. (p. 1)

The 1998 Green Paper was the first major educational policy document to emerge from the then newly elected Labour Government and it proposed not only major reforms around pay and careers, but also to turn teaching into 'a first class profession'. The then Secretary of State for Education, David Blunkett believed that the Green Paper proposals would create

> ... a new vision of the profession which offers better rewards and support in return for higher standards. (DfEE, 1998b)

The Green Paper received a great deal of publicity and prompted a lot of public debate about the status of teachers and teaching, not least among teachers and their professional organisations among whom it was initially not well received (Bricheno & Thornton, 1999). However, with hindsight, we can see that the Green Paper proposals did result in a step change in teacher salaries, careers and working conditions.

Teachers now have rights to non-contact time to undertake planning, preparation, and assessment (PPA) and have been released from a range of clerical and 'non-teaching' tasks as part of the workforce reforms (DES, 2003). There has been a mass expansion in the numbers of classroom assistants (again initially resisted by teacher unions), and Higher Level Teaching Assistants (HLTAs), qualified through additional training, working closely with teachers, undertaking teaching and learning activities with small groups and whole classes in the teachers' absence.

The programme of reform and investment to raise the status of teachers and the teaching profession, undertaken by the Labour Government, appears to have been successful, despite including the introduction of performance-related pay, changes to the curriculum and a constant flow of new educational initiatives. There appears to have been a profound turnaround in the way in which teachers are perceived by politicians and are presented to the public.

Changing perceptions of male primary teachers

Current government policy, and much of the media reporting of education, suggests that male primary/early-years teachers have something unique and positive to offer young children—their gender. They are considered desirable because they can act as 'positive role models for boys' (DfEE, 1998a, p. 225). Such changes in Government policy are in line with public opinion, with parents now far more willing to accept men working with young children (Hinsliff, 2003) and less concern about men being potentially dangerous to them (Owen, 2003; Sargent, 2005).

The high profile scrutiny of male teachers appears to have lessened somewhat between 1998 and 2005. Headlines such as 'Pervert label puts men off teaching' (Budge, 1998, p. 1), 'Male teachers fear slurs' (Carvel, 1998, p. 2) and 'An unsuitable job for a man' (Furedi, 2000, p. 5) are now much rarer. Men may also have benefited from greater public awareness of their rarity, and through arguments and increasingly prevalent assertions about their value and importance in teaching, especially as role models for boys.

Between 1998 and 2005, there were frequent calls for more male teachers to act as 'positive role models for boys'. It was a 'National Priority' according to *The Guardian* (2002), while Lepkowska, in *The Express* (2000), pleaded 'Please Sir, our young pupils need your skills'. In 2000, Secretary of State for Education, David Blunkett said 'We need more good male role models to challenge boys' resistance to learning and laddish behaviour' (DfEE, 2000). School standards minister, Stephen Timms (Woodward, 2002) said it was 'important that boys in primary schools had male role models', while Diane Abbott MP claimed the problem of black male underachievement in school was partly due to the preponderance of white female teachers (Merrick, 2002). In 2002, the Teacher Training agency introduced targets for recruiting more men to train for primary teaching, while in 2005 Liam Fox, then Conservative Shadow Minister for Education, suggested that 'boys should be taught in single-sex schools with strong male role models to help a lost generation of fatherless young men find their way in life' (Hinsliff & Temko, 2005).

These well-publicised statements, which contributed to the myth (Thornton & Bricheno, 2006) that male teachers automatically instil better discipline and enhance boys achievements, may well have served to raise perceptions about the status of male teachers, while possibly, at the same time, lowering that of women teachers (TES, 2002). Taken together with Government policy changes since 1997, which have clearly been successful in terms of improving teachers' pay and status and have addressed workload issues, it would seem that the balance between disincentives and incentives to men teaching young children may have changed between 1998 and 2005.

Conclusions

This article has explored the differences between 1998 entrants concerns about teaching and those of leavers in 2005. That there are differences between them we have no doubt. However, what might have caused these differences is subject to speculation. We have suggested that one possible explanation for the differences might lie in social and political changes that took place between 1998 and 2005, namely a change in the ways in which teachers and their status were presented in the media and how they were viewed and treated by two different governments—the Conservatives up to 1997 and the New Labour (to date).

Men are more likely than women to leave teaching for higher pay and better opportunities elsewhere, and this is especially true for men in primary teaching (Thornton & Bricheno, 2006, p. 139). Male teachers, particularly male primary teachers, have a choice of better paid options open to them. But there are some strong indications that the image of teachers presented in the news media, and public and teachers own perceptions of their status, improved between 1998 and 2005. Concerns about male teachers being perceived as gay or paedophilic appear to have lessened somewhat. The expressed concerns of teachers now are different from what they were in 1998, and this may mark a turning point for the numbers of men in primary teaching.

However, there remain two over-riding concerns for teachers: the intense government interference that some believe erodes their professionalism, and the issue of pupils' poor behaviour. Both appear to be more important to men than to women, and may continue to act as disincentives to men becoming primary teachers.

References

Alexander, R., Rose, J. & Woodhead, C. (1992) *Curriculum organisation and classroom practice in primary schools: a discussion paper* (London, DES).

Barmby, P. & Coe, R. (2004) Recruiting and retaining teachers: findings from recent studies, paper presented at the *British Educational Research Association Conference*, Manchester, 14–18 September.

Bricheno, P. & Thornton, M. (1999) Credentialism and structure in primary teachers' careers, paper presented at the *British Educational Research Association Conference*, University of Sussex, September.

Budge, D. (1998, August 28) Pervert label puts men off teaching, *Times Educational Supplement*, p. 1.

Carrington, B. (2002) A quintessentially feminine domain? Student teachers' constructions of primary teaching as a career, *Educational Studies*, 28(3), 287–303.

Carvel, J. (1998, August 29) Male teachers fear slurs, *The Guardian*, p. 2.

Cockburn, C. (1991) *In the way of women: men's resistance to sex equality in organizations* (London, Macmillan).

Dolton, P. & Chung, T.-P. (2004) The rate of return to teaching: how does it compare to other graduate jobs, *National Institute Economic Review, 190*, 89–103.

DES (1989) *The Education Reform Act 1988: the school curriculum and assessment* (Circular no. 5/89) (London, HMSO).

DES (2003) *Raising standards and tackling workload: a national agreement on workforce reform— taking forward the school workforce reforms.* Available online at: http://www.governornet.co.uk/cropArticle.cfm?topicAreaId=4&contentId=515&mode=bg (accessed 30 October 2007).

DfEE (1998a) *Meeting the childcare challenge: a framework consultation document.* (White Paper) (London: The Stationery Office) (Department for Social Security and Ministers for Women).

DfEE (1998b) *Meeting the childcare challenge: a framework consultation document.* (Green Paper) (London, The Stationery Office).

DfEE (2000, August 20) *Boys must improve at same rate as girls* (D. Blunkett, Press Notice 2000/0368). Available online at: http://www.dfes.gov.uk/pns/DisplayPN.cgi?pn_id=2000_0368 (accessed 7 August 2008).

Drudy, S., Martin, M., Woods, M. & O'Flynn, J. (2005) *Men and the classroom: gender imbalances in teaching* (London, RoutledgeFalmer).

Furedi, F. (2000, October 12) An unsuitable job for a man, *The Independent*, p. 5.

Hargreaves, L., Cunningham, M., Everton, T., *et al.* (2007) *The status of teachers and the teaching profession in England: views from inside and outside the profession.* Evidence Base. Research Report RR831B (London, DfES).

Haughton, E. (2002, February 28) Men: your classroom needs you, *The Independent*.

Hinsliff, G. (2003, June 8) Men battle prejudice in childcare, *The Observer*. Available online at: http://education.guardian.co.uk/schools/story/0,,973651,00.html (accessed 7 August 2008).

Hinsliff, G. & Temko, N. (2005, July 3) Fox calls for single-sex schools, *The Observer*.

Hobson, A. J. & Malderez, A. (Eds) with Kerr, K., Tracey, L., Pell, R. G., *et al.* (2005) *Becoming a teacher: student teachers' motives and preconceptions, and early school-based experiences during Initial Teacher Training (ITT).* DfES Research Report No. 673.

House of Commons Education and Skills Committee (2004) *Secondary education: teacher retention and recruitment.* Fifth Report of Session 2003–04, Vols. I and II, HC 1057-1 and HC 1057-11 (London, Stationery Office).

Johnston, J., McKeown, E. & McEwen, A. (1999) Choosing primary teaching as a career: the perspectives of males and females in training, *Journal of Education for Teaching, 25*(1), 55–64.

Lepkowska, D. (2000, January 31) Please sir, our young pupils need your skills, *The Express* (Micro Edition).

Mac an Ghaill, M. (1994) *The making of men: masculinities, sexualities and schooling* (Buckingham, Open University Press).

Merrick, J. (2002, January 7) Black boys' need more male teachers, *Times Educational Supplement*.

Mills, M. (2005) The male teacher debate Australian style: the Catholic Education Office (CEO) vs Human Rights and Equal Opportunities Commission (HREOC), paper presented at the *Graduate School of Education*, Queen's University, Belfast, 6 May.

Morris, E. (2001) Professionalism and trust, a speech to the Social Market Foundation, London, DES, 12 November.

Owen, C. (2003) *Men's work? Changing the gender mix of the childcare and early years workforce* (Facing the Future: Policy Papers 6) (London, Day Care Trust).

Pringle, K. (1998) Men as workers in professional childcare settings: an anti-oppressive practice framework, in: C. Owen, C. Cameron & P. Moss (Eds) *Men as workers in services for young children: issues of a mixed gender workforce* (Bedford Way Papers) (London, Institute of Education, University of London), 163–181.

Reid, I. & Thornton, M. (2000) *Students' reasons for choosing primary teaching as a career* (Aldenham, Centre for Equality Issues in Education, University of Hertfordshire).

Sargent, P. (2005) The gendering of men in early childhood education, *Sex Roles, 52*(3–4), 251–259.

Smedley, S. (1999) Don't rock the boat: men student teachers' understanding of gender and equality, paper presented at the *British Educational Research Association Conference*, University of Sussex, September.

Smithers, A. & Robinson, P. (2004) *Teacher turnover, wastage and destinations.* Research Report 553 (London, DfES).

Spear, M., Gould, K. & Lee, B. (2000) *Who would be a teacher? A review of factors motivating and demotivating prospective and practising teachers* (Slough, National Foundation for Educational Research).

Sturman, L. (2002) *Contented and committed? A survey of quality of working life amongst teachers* (Slough, National Foundation for Educational Research).

TES (2002, September 13) Man trouble, *Times Educational Supplement* (Editorial).

Thornton, M. (2001) Men, pre-service training and the implications for continuing professional development, *Journal of In-service Education*, 27(3), 477–490.

Thornton, M. & Bricheno, P. (2006) *Missing men in education* (Stoke-on-Trent, Trentham Books).

Whitehead, S. M. (2002) *Men and masculinities* (Cambridge, Polity).

Woodward, W. (2002, August 22) The drive to recruit male primary teachers, *The Guardian*.

New Zealand men's participation in early years work[1]

Sarah-Eve Farquhar

Childforum Research, New Zealand

The New Zealand context

As a world leader in women's suffrage, New Zealand has an international image as a trial-blazing 'social laboratory'. In 1893 women were granted the right to vote in parliamentary elections. Britain and the USA among most other democracies did not give women the right to vote until after World War I. In politics today 33% of New Zealand's parliamentarians are women. Women, not men, recently held all the key constitutional positions of Prime Minister, Governor General, Speaker of the House of Representatives and Chief Justice. Women's participation in paid employment is high—women make up 46.1% of the country's labour force (National Equal Opportunities Network, 2008).

However, there are several indicators that equality for women in employment still has far to go. First, the hourly earnings of women are about 85% of men's hourly pay pack. Member of Parliament Ruth Dyson (2007) explained that 85% sounds good but the pay gap between women and men has moved little in the last 20 years (by only about 0.4% per year). Second, in the boardrooms and in traditionally male occupations where there is now greater female representation, such as in the police, journalism, law and in the universities, men still hold most of the senior positions. Third, the majority of women are clustered in traditionally female occupations, such as nursing and early childcare teaching.

The problem, I wish to argue here, is that the success of our 'social laboratory' has been limited by focusing almost exclusively on women's disadvantage and largely ignoring areas of disadvantage for men. Further, this limited success has impacted not only on women and men but on children also and the quality of family life. For example, a Ministry of Social Development (2006) survey reported that 35% of families with both parents in paid work would prefer one parent to stay home if they could financially afford to. Current government policy positions women as needing more paid work (still) and promotes greater marketisation of childcare responsibilities (Kahu & Morgan, 2008).

In this paper, I look specifically at changes in the male and female workforce in childcare and teaching. This is an occupation that has become more, and not less, entrenched as a women's occupation. It has implications for:

- women's achievement of equality in the wider labour force;
- men's choices to engage in non-traditional work and have the opportunity, like women, to work with children in childcare and education;
- children whose potential opportunities for contact with nurturing male adults are reduced the longer they spend in early childcare and education;
- dads to feel welcome and comfortable about entering the early childcare setting and being involved with children within the female dominated setting, and
- the number and range of potential employees that employers have to choose from and their ability to get the best childcare teachers for their service.

In 1992 around 2.34% of the childcare teaching workforce was male, but male representation has steadily slipped since the early 1990s to just less than 1%. Across the Tasman, Australian males have a reputation for being 'macho', and of being very sexist towards women. It should be an embarrassment to us in New Zealand that Australia has a much higher male participation rate in childcare teaching—about two to four times higher. However, it's been a point of pride, not shame, that the early childhood workforce is dominated by women (e.g. see Meade, 1990; Duncan & Rowe, 1997; May, 2001).

Surprisingly, the dearth of men in childcare teaching is at odds with greater father involvement with children's care in the private sphere of the home (Callister, 1999). Because of New Zealand's high female participation rate in paid employment, female partners or wives require or depend on support from their male partners or husbands (McPherson, 2006). Further, in New Zealand society it is now considered 'cool' to be an involved dad and men themselves want to be more involved. Surprisingly also, as the size of the childcare teaching workforce has expanded to more than double over the past 10–15 years, the actual number of male childcare teaching staff has dropped. In this paper the reasons for a decline in male representation in childcare teaching are outlined, along with the challenges involved and recent changes.

Sex abuse paranoia

Unlike other traditionally female occupations whose male participation rates have either stayed much the same or have increased over the past decade, childcare teaching stands out as the one that has suffered a decline. For example, male registered nurses make up 6.5% of the nursing and midwifery workforce, and around 33% of flight attendants are male (Farquhar *et al.*, 2006).

The decline in male participation relative to women's in childcare teaching started after a sex abuse case, initially involving a male childcare worker and a number of female co-workers at a South Island City Council 'Civic Childcare Centre'. The case resulted in the conviction of childcare teacher Peter Ellis for 10 years in 1993 and had an enormous negative effect on public perception of the safety of children in centres. A further case appeared before the courts from a North Island hospital crèche resulting in Geoffrey Scott being jailed for seven years in 1994. While these cases created difficulty for women working in childcare teaching, the paranoia around child sex abuse was most strongly felt by men in both the South and the North Islands of New Zealand. It negatively affected the personal confidence of men already working in childcare teaching and those considering this work, as the following quotations from Farquhar (1997a) illustrate:

Irene: Before the abuse cases came up things were different, it was exciting. People would ring up or come around and look and say 'wow, you've got a male staff member, how wonderful!' (p. 29)

Martin: [My mother] keeps telling me to get out. She is trying to protect me from the stigma, from any sort of accusation. (p. 21)

Denis: On my first day in my first job there was a lot of difficulty in the kindergarten and some parents left because I was appointed there. No one had met me. It was partly because they weren't sure after the Civic situation. (p. 31)

Martin: I have been assaulted because I am a male early childhood worker. An acquaintance of one of my ex-flatmates, her brother came back to Wellington from Australia just as the hospital crèche case was going to court … I had never met him. He came around to the door with a name tag on his shirt and said he was doing a survey, and asked what I did. I said 'childcare worker', and he just burst into the house and started beating me up. He was saying 'I know what you are doing'. (p. 31)

Ivan: Even for boys I am not doing as much [nappy and clothes] changing as I used to do. It's something that the female teachers often just volunteer to do the changing. I think they realise the situation now. (p. 33)

Hayley: Doug I know feels difficult about cuddling a child, which is really sad. He still does cuddle them, but he's very aware of what the outcome could be. (p. 32)

Desmond: There was a staff member who accidently scraped a child's penis with her fingernail, and what if that child had told his parents? If there was any suspicion people would instinctively think of me more than the female staff. I have to be more careful than the other staff. (p. 30)

The Ministry of Education (1993) acted calmly to educate childcare teachers on strategies to keep children safe from sex abuse through the publication of guidelines. This was widely taken up and used by centre managers and teachers to reassure parents that centres had learnt from these cases and that procedures were now in place to ensure children's safety. Male teachers, however, really needed support and someone to speak up for them. Education Minister, Wyatt Creech, acknowledged that male teachers faced the possibility of over-reaction about child sex abuse issues even though such problems were rare. 'It's obviously a concern because we would like to see more gender balance in the early childhood profession and in teaching generally' (reported in Tocker, 1997). However he viewed that little else, apart from publication of the Ministry of Education (1993) guidelines, could be done about this because it came down to public attitudes.

Male childcare teachers were left unsupported by professional bodies and leaders who perhaps were themselves too afraid or felt it too un-politically correct to speak out in defence of the participation of men in teaching. Union national secretary Joanna Beresford rejected the possibility and Farquhar's (1997a) research that sex abuse fears were having an effect on male childcare teachers and on the willingness of men to enter the profession.

> 'If you found early childhood workers were going to be paid $50,000 a year, you'd suddenly have lots of men seeking to train', she said … 'While a few male teachers had reported not being fully trusted in their work after the Ellis case, the concerns appeared to have died off', Ms Beresford said. (reported in Tocker, 1997)

The early childhood and primary school teachers' union NZEI Te Riu Roa went so far as to promote fear by telling teachers not to touch children because any form of touch could be misconstrued as child abuse. It seemed to be in the union's best interests to do this. Teachers became dependent on the union as their representatives to help them to deal with this growing paranoia and to assist them with employment issues and legal processes. NZEI Te Riu Roa's (1988, updated) *Code of Conduct* was written for teachers in primary schools and not specifically for childcare teachers, but as nearly all childcare teachers belonged to the union the *Code* influenced their thinking and the views and expectations of teacher educators and others in the profession. Union national secretary, Joanna Beresford said:

> … teachers were advised not to touch children, except when absolutely necessary, and then only if another adult was present. It is regrettable that has to be our advice. We have had instances where completely innocent actions have been misconstrued. (Morgan, 1999, p. 3)

It has been argued that NZEI's recommendations and responses served to fuel public concerns rather than sending out a message that teachers were professionals and such cases of sex abuse were rare. What resulted has been described as a 'moral panic' around teachers' relationship with children, with negative outcomes for male teachers in particular, and for children (see Farquhar, 2001). However, the union issued a press release critical of this view and arguing that it was an overstatement (NZEI, 1999).

Well over a decade since these two childcare centre abuse cases, with no further such prosecutions of men in childcare teaching and after strong doubt has been placed on the correctness of the conviction of Peter Ellis (Hood, 2001), male childcare teachers just want this issue to go away (Farquhar, 2007). It will help that the union has recently replaced the *Code of Conduct* with a short guideline statement for both childcare and primary teachers stating that touch is okay in certain situations and circumstances (NZEI, 2006). However, after such a long period of little positive action and little speaking up on behalf and in support of male teachers, bringing male participation rates back up to the early 1990s level of 2.4% will take more than recognition that child sex abuse fears should not be used to keep men out of childcare teaching. Not withstanding the sex abuse issue, there are also other reasons for the low male participation level in childcare teaching in New Zealand as discussed in the sections below.

Questioning men's masculinity, ability and right to be childcare teachers

There is room for improvement in New Zealand's 'social laboratory' that sees women's disadvantage as a problem for society, but men's disadvantage as a problem for individual men (Callister, 2007). If government policies focused on men's rights and employment opportunities as well as women's then men in childcare teaching would not be left essentially on their own to try to counter stereotypes and to 'prove' their ability. This gender bias in government policies has created a situation in which men who are in childcare teaching have to be, and are, 'superheroes':

> I would like to share a comment I received by way of a card today. 'We think only a super-hero decides to be a kindy teacher'. That in itself sums up the importance of males in early childhood. Look at that guys, we are superheroes. I think I might leave the tights at home though. (Neill, 2007, p. 47)

Male childcare teachers can face questions and unwelcomed assumptions about their sexuality, for example:

> Doug: Being a person who has always been in a relationship, or in an active heterosexual relationship right the way through and having children of my own has helped people find out fairly soon and to realise 'oh well, he can't be gay'.
>
> Noel: In 1991 a family came into the kindergarten. Towards the end of the morning the child's mother came up to me and asked if she could have a word with me … She was asking questions on behalf of her husband. They wanted to know if I was a practising homosexual. (Farquhar, 1997b, p. 412)

Their ability to be childcare teachers can be overlooked and mean that men are not advised of childcare teaching as a career option.

> May: The high schools don't encourage young men to come for work experience. I can't believe that out of the two big high schools here that there wouldn't be one boy who would be interested. (Farquhar, 1997a, p. 22)

Men's ability to be childcare teachers can be questioned within the profession. But, women who have experienced working with a male colleague tend to think otherwise. Even so, men can still feel social/professional pressure to prove their competency particularly in the area of domestic tasks (Farquhar, 1997a).

Don: There is a fraction of women teachers who don't want men. They say they can do the job fine without men. I've found this in the union, particularly with the stronger women who say that we don't need men in early childhood. (p. 25)

Glen: It's like a coloured person walking into an all-white club. You are going to be discriminated against because women, if they have their own personal agenda, will work together, to exclude men. (p. 24)

Roxanne: I've had to learn that men are just as good, they just look at things differently and they do things differently from women. Because it is largely women who run the show they (other women) don't see that what men do is always right. (p. 22)

Elle: He is really good in the family play. He gets dressed up. He's really active and vital. The kids get such a kick out of playing with him and they will hang around him for company. (p. 37)

Len: They pick on you like 'Len doesn't like doing the dishes' ... I then have to prove that I do the dishes. They can get away with not doing the dishes. (p. 28)

Because lack of participation in childcare teaching has been viewed as a problem for individual men to get on and cope with, male teachers can feel isolated and often alone. For example:

I have kept in touch with many of my former students. It is tough for the men to stay in teaching, not because of the work but because of the attitudes of female staff. One Chinese guy has been working in a centre for just under a year and he tells me that although he enjoys working with children, he often feels lonely ... Basically the women don't include him in their casual conversations and he feels quite 'left out'. (Heald, 2007, p. 43)

Men who have a strong sense of identity and come into teaching after having other work experiences are perhaps more able to understand and cope with reactions and expectations towards themselves as males within a female-dominated women's occupation (Buckingham *et al.*, 2007).

Challenges and changes

A sudden change in outlook

Farquhar's (1997a) small study of the views and experiences of 20 male and 20 female childcare and kindergarten teachers was picked up by, and discussed widely within, the television, print and radio media. This media attention stimulated public awareness of the downward trend in male participation in teaching and to calls for children to have positive male role models in the early years. The problem of fewer male teachers has continued to be raised often in the media since, and not just for childcare teaching but also now for primary and secondary teaching. But media interest and public concern was mostly ignored by those in official and professional circles who could have made change. Childcare teaching was considered to be a good source of employment for women needing or wanting to get back into paid work and looking for a second chance career. Women were available to fill positions as the profession grew and expanded, and any targeting or advertising promotions for men would have been seen to be detrimental to the employment opportunities of women. As well, the sex abuse issue was one that those in official and professional circles did not seem to want to tackle so it was easier to do nothing.

Years later, Adam Buckingham sent copies of work he had done for a university assignment and a presentation on the importance of men in childcare teaching to me (Sarah-Eve Farquhar). I read this and suggested to Adam that perhaps it was time to put something into print again. So at the end of 2005/early 2006 I wrote to three other men working at different levels and with different experiences in childcare teaching and suggested we put together a paper to update the situation since the initial research report of 1997. By chance a reporter, with whom I shared a copy of our draft report with, was now working as a field producer for Television New Zealand (TVNZ); and that very same day we were told that they would be very interested in making a documentary and requested to delay releasing the report until then. Making and then finally screening the documentary 'A Few Good Men' (TVNZ, 2006) took many months, especially as each Sunday when we thought the documentary would be screened another important national or international event, such as the death of Crocodile Man Steve Irwin, would come up. However, the time lag between the completion of our report and the documentary screening gave the Minister of Education, his staff in the Ministry and others, who had been interviewed or talked with as part of making the documentary but were not necessarily shown on it, time to think and time to initiate some action.

The Early Childhood Council, which represents the majority of private and community childcare services in New Zealand, issued a press release immediately after the screening of the TVNZ documentary saying that the lack of men in childcare teaching was 'a national disgrace'. The Early Childhood Council in taking a stand on this issue and in organising its 2007 Conference on the theme of men in early childhood education showed leadership. The Council along with competing early childhood organisations found the issue to be one that they could talk about and together on. Importantly, male early childhood teachers have formed a support network; and because of the changed professional and political climate they are willing to put themselves out and promote the importance of their role as teachers of young children (see www.ecmenz.org). A number of organisations, including the National Equal Opportunities Network (2007) carried articles about the First Summit for Men in Early Childcare and Teaching, and a second very successful Summit bringing male teachers from across New Zealand together was held this year (2008).

Pay, professionalism and status

The professionalisation of the childcare teaching workforce went hand in hand with cementing the centrality of women as childcare teachers. Belgium researcher, Peeters

(2007), makes the point that a 'high level of professionalism does not automatically lead to a mixed-gender workforce' (p. 17). This is true of the situation in childcare teaching in New Zealand. As the size of the workforce has expanded, the representation of men has decreased. In contrast, the participation of men is stronger than ever in services staffed by non-professionals (parents), such as Playcentres (services that provide parent education and training for parents) and Nga Kohanga Reo (Maori language centres that involve parents in children's learning).

Today childcare teaching is not a low-pay low-status occupation. It has, in recent years, become a financially attractive career choice. From July 2002 pay parity with primary teachers was phased in for kindergarten teachers, and this influences and benefits the employment contracts of childcare teachers in other early years services. Services that employ diploma/degree qualified staff are given a significantly higher level of hourly funding per child by the government and so services are able to pay the higher costs of qualified staff.

In most parts of New Zealand there is a moderate to severe shortage of childcare teachers, which creates the perfect climate for childcare teachers to seek out the highest paying positions and to negotiate a higher wage. For example, in the biggest city of Auckland there is a severe shortage.

> Demand has outweighed supply for a long time in city centres, with reports of some parents trying to book places for children who were not yet conceived. But the [government's] Working for Families policy and the free [childcare] hours scheme have enabled—and put pressure on—more people to return to work, adding to the squeeze at childcare centres ... Barriers to increasing daycare provision is a shortage of trained staff and a Government ruling that centres must have at least 50 per cent qualified staff. A spokeswoman for daycare provider Kindercares, Barbar Tozer, says some centres have advertised for staff repeatedly without receiving a single application. One Montessori centre in Matakana has been advertising for a teacher since the beginning of the year. (Jones, 2008)

The government's Career Services (2004–2008) explains that the shortages (called 'employment opportunities') are primarily due to new government policy which has:

- provided a definition of a qualified childcare teacher;
- specified that services must have teaching diploma/degree staff on-site at all times and that by 2012 all staff must hold a diploma or be in training;
- highlighted the educational benefits of childcare facilities to encourage parental use for children;
- encouraged parents to return after 14 weeks parental leave through childcare allowances; and
- provided funding of 20 hours free childcare in services staffed by professional teachers for all three- and four-year olds to increase children's hours of participation and increase employment opportunities for trained childcare teachers.

It seems that the pragmatics of a shortage of childcare teachers today is the one reason why suddenly it has gone from being politically incorrect to speak of needing men in childcare teaching to being politically correct. Men are a potential untapped pool of labour. This is the argument for getting more men into childcare teaching that has won through. The TVNZ documentary probably would not have led to anything had it not come just at the time when government was struggling with how it would meet its policy goals for early childhood education and when employers were getting increasingly worried about how they could comply with government demands around staffing. Further, it's now possible for professional and governmental organisations to take up the issue of a lack of male childcare teachers without fear of offending women or being seen to put children at risk of being abused. The hysteria that surrounded the sex abuse cases during the 1990s and for so many years was fuelled by teachers being told by their union that they could be accused of abuse at any time, has died down although obviously the effects of the hysteria are still being felt.

Thus, government agencies are now motivated to portray men in promotional materials and redefine childcare teaching as a profession for men and women. As well, the teachers' union has deleted or removed links to its website pages stating that it is proud that 75% of its membership was female and highlighting the central role of its Women's Network, and it now includes a page on men in teaching. However, it remains to be seen whether this will all spill over to such things as how equal employment opportunity (EEO) policy is applied to the childcare teaching situation. For example, the 2006–07 Collective Agreement, between the union and the state services commission for kindergarten teachers, head teachers and senior teachers did not mention the employment requirements of men but did include a section on good employer practice which listed a responsibility to recognise the employment requirements of women.

Institutionalised sexism

Even though there is now emerging acceptance at official and professional levels that there is a place for men in childcare teaching, institutionalised sexism may be a barrier that will take a lot longer to change, as this story from a male childcare teacher illustrates:

> I came home one day to my foster daughter screaming to me that there was a dead mouse floating in her fishbowl. As it had been an interesting week I looked at this poor wee soul and thought 'I know how you feel, mate'. At times this is so true through the often isolated professional work place, the gender imbalances that dominate our lives as men in early childhood through to the often feminisation of the education system itself, we can feel like a mouse invading an environment that historically we could have stayed well clear off. (Neill, 2007, p. 42)

Within and between the intersections of recruitment, training and graduation those problems can exist for men in becoming childcare teachers.

> You will be interested to hear that I was approached by a hopeful male trainee teacher last week who read the story about our teacher [name of male teacher deleted] in something from TeachNZ (he said). [TeachNZ is a government agency that is responsible for teacher recruitment and promotion.] He knocked on the door and introduced himself and said the

article gave him the confidence to approach us. It sounds like he has lots of knock backs in both primary and early childhood education in NZ. (personal communication from an Auckland childcare centre manager, March 2008)

Because there are so few men in childcare teaching, men considering becoming a childcare teacher rarely have contact with other male teachers and with men who can support them through the application process and training. This is seen to be a major disadvantage, resulting in men not being successful in the application process and dropping out of teacher training. At the first Summit for men in childcare teaching a number of recommendations to help address sexism and support male participation during recruitment, training and employment were put forward (Farquhar, 2007). Most of the recommendations centred on problems associated with:

- the way childcare teaching was portrayed and promoted;
- recruitment and open days being run, or presented, by women and not by men also;
- biases against men within teacher education course content;
- financial strains for men taking up three-year training including difficulty of accessing teaching scholarships and lack of availability of one-year graduate programmes; and
- lack of recognition that men are more likely to stay in training and in employment if they are not segregated from other men (pp. 8–9).

Conclusion

The New Zealand experience highlights that it is possible to keep talking and advocating for men in childcare teaching until the 'cow's come home' (a common kiwi expression). For any real shift in sexist attitudes and for the door to be opened to men as widely as it is for women, a necessity needs to be present or created. In New Zealand this necessity is that there is a staffing shortage which is hindering the profession from moving more quickly to being an all teacher-qualified workforce, and hindering the realisation of government goals to increase children's participation in non-parental care and encourage parents to participate in greater amounts of paid work.

At last, New Zealand's international image as a trail-blazing social laboratory for women may be renewed if the gender bias that exists in childcare teaching is successfully addressed. It remains to be seen, however, whether childcare teaching will continue to reproduce its own patterns of recruitment, training and working environments, or whether a more male-friendly culture will emerge (Peeters, 2007). Much may depend too, on the policies of the next and future governments, as the Education Minister has significant influence over the early years education sector, unlike the pre-1990s when government had little influence over the characteristics of the workforce. There is also a question that is yet to be asked as to whether it is a good thing that the main impetus for the sudden interest in male participation in childcare teaching is a labour shortage. On average New Zealanders already work longer hours per week than people in most other developed countries, and government policy aimed at raising the amount of time that children spend in childcare/early childhood education may not necessarily be desirable for all children and their contact with their fathers, mothers and participation in community life—but this is another paper.

Note

1.   For further papers and NZ research on this topic, see http://www.childforum.com.

References

Buckingham, A., Cottom, S., Fisher, D. & Armstrong, G. (2007) Avoiding the minefield as a male in teacher training and employment: tips and strategies for survival, in: S.-E. Farquhar (Ed) *Proceedings of the first New Zealand Men in Early Child Care and Teaching Summit and a Record of Challenges, Changes and Thinking* (Wellington, Childforum Research), 30–33.

Callister, P. (1999) Iron John or ironing John? The changing lives of New Zealand fathers, in: S. Birks & P. Callister (Eds) *Perspectives on fathering. Issues Paper No. 4* (Palmerston North, Massey University). Available online at: http://econ.massey.ac.nz/cppe/papers/cppeip04/cppeip4c.pdf (accessed 4 April 2008).

Callister, P. (2007) Gender and tertiary education, in: S. Farquhar (Ed) *Proceedings of the first NZ Men in Early Child Care and Teaching Summit* (Porirua, NZ: Childforum), 23–29.

Career Services. (variously dated pages 2004–2008) *Early childhood teacher.* Available online at: http://www.careers.govt.nz/default.aspx?id0=60103&id1=J35420 (accessed 4 April 2008).

Duncan, J., & Rowe, L. (1997) Don't be too polite girls, don't be too polite: kindergarten teachers and employment contracts, *New Zealand Annual Review of Education 1996*, 5, 157–180.

Dyson, R. (2007, 27 February) *Address to Pay and Employment Equity Forum.* Speech notes (Wellington, Town Hall).

Farquhar, S.-E. (1997a) *A few good men or a few too many? A study of male teachers* (Palmerston North, Massey University).

Farquhar, S.-E. (1997b) Of puppy dog tails, sugar and spice: gender inequality and discrimination in early childhood education, *Delta*, 49(2), 405–416.

Farquhar, S.-E. (2001) Moral panic in New Zealand: teachers touching children, in: A. Jones (Ed) *Touchy subject: teachers touching children* (Dunedin, University of Otago Press), 87–98.

Farquhar, S.-E. (Ed) (2007) *Proceedings of the first New Zealand Men in Early Child Care and Teaching Summit and a Record of Challenges, Changes and Thinking* (Wellington, Childforum Research).

Farquhar, S.-E., Cablk, L., Buckingham, A., Butler, D. & Ballantyne, D. (2006) *Men at work: sexism in early childhood education* (Wellington, Childforum Research).

Heald, D. (2007) Attracting men into early childhood work, in: S. Farquhar (Ed) *Proceedings of the first New Zealand Men in Early Child Care and Teaching Summit and a Record of Challenges, Changes and Thinking* (Wellington, Childforum Research), 43.

Hood, L. (2001) *A city possessed: the Christchurch civic crèche case* (Dunedin, Longacre Press).

Jones, M. (2008, March 16) Parents struggle to find childcare places, *New Zealand Herald.* Available online at: http://www.nzherald.co.nz/section/1/story.cfm?c_id=1&objectid=10498427 (accessed 4 April 2008).

Kahu, E. R. & Morgan, M. (2008) Making choices: contradictions and commonalities in the valuing of caring and working by government policy and first time mothers, *New Zealand Research in Early Childhood Education*, 11, 1–18.

May, H. (2001) *Politics in the playground: the world of early childhood in postwar New Zealand* (Wellington, Bridget Williams Books and NZCER).

McPherson, M. (2006) *NZ cultural norms of parenting and childcare and how these relate to labour force participation decisions and requirements* (Wellington, Families Commission).

Meade, A. (1990) Women and children gain a foot in the door, *Women's Studies Journal*, 6(1), 38–46.

Ministry of Education (1993) *Prevent child abuse: guidelines for early childhood services* (Wellington, Learning Media).

Ministry of Social Development (2006) *Work, family and parenting study: research findings.* Available online at: http://www.msd.govt.nz/work-areas/social-research/families-whanau/work-family-and-parenting.html (accessed 5 February 2008).

Morgan, J. (1999, November 9) Teachers should touch children: lecturer, *The Dominion*, p. 3.

National Equal Opportunities Network (2007) *Why do we need men in early childhood education?* Available online at: http://www.neon.org.nz/newsarchive/meninearlychildhoodeducation/ (accessed 4 April 2008).

National Equal Opportunities Network (2008) *New Zealand census of women's participation, 2008* (Wellington, Author).

Neill, D. (2007) A mouse in a fishbowl, in: S. Farquhar (Ed) *Proceedings of the first New Zealand Men in Early Child Care and Teaching Summit and a Record of Challenges, Changes and Thinking* (Wellington, Childforum Research), 42.

NZEI (1999) *NZEI advocates common sense in caring for children* (Press release, 10 November).

NZEI (2006) *Guidelines: physical contact with children.* Available online at: http://www.nzei.org.nz/annual_meeting/annual_meeting06/documents/GuidelinesPhysical.pdf (accessed 4 April 2008).

NZEI Te Riu Roa. (1998, updated) *Service and support staff manual—schools. Code of conduct: physical contact with children* (Wellington, Author).

Peeters, J. (2007) Including men in early childhood education: insights from the European experience, *NZ Research in ECE*, 10, 15–24.

Tocker, A. (1997, January 28) Men scared off teaching by sex claims: report, *The Dominion*. http://www.peterellis.org.nz/1997/1997-0128_Dominion_MenScaredOffTeachingBySexClaimsReport.htm

TVNZ (Television New Zealand). (2006) *A few good men: a documentary on the 'Sunday' programme, 24 September.* Available online at: http://tvnz.co.nz/view/video_popup_windows_skin/835057 (accessed 3 March 2008).

Father involvement in early childhood programs: review of the literature

Glen Palm[a] and Jay Fagan[b]

[a]Child & Family Studies, St. Cloud State University, USA; [b]School of Social Administration, Temple University, USA

Fathers in early childhood programs

Father involvement in early childhood programs (ECPs) has increased over the last 10–15 years supported by recent attention on the positive influences of fathers on children (e.g., Pruett, 2000; Lewis & Lamb, 2004). Program initiatives such as Early Head Start (EHS) (Cabrera, 2004), and the fact that the majority of children ages 0–5 are enrolled in one or more programs in the USA make ECPs an important context for engaging fathers and supporting positive father involvement (Fagan & Palm, 2004; McBride & Lutz, 2004). This review of our understanding of the current state of father involvement in ECPs will employ two different theoretical frameworks: an ecological perspective (Fagan, 1999) and a more narrow focus of situated fathering

(Marsiglio *et al.*, 2005). The purpose of this review of research and practice literature is to understand the current levels of father involvement in early education programs, the factors that support this type of father involvement, the barriers to father involvement, and strategies for increasing father involvement in ECPs.

Defining fathers and father involvement in ECPs

The review of this topic has to begin with some clarification about the definition of fatherhood. In a recent publication (MFFN, 2007), the definition of fatherhood was addressed as a complex reality that has led to more than a dozen different definitions of fathers that reflect changing family contexts and realities. These definitions include biological connections, social connections, legal connections and psychological presence. The focus of most research continues to be on the biological father and most often in the two-parent family. However, there have been recent attempts to understand the role of unmarried and nonresidential fathers in the lives of young children (Fragile Families and Child Wellbeing research, e.g., McLanahan & Carlson, 2004). This research confirms that fathers represent a diverse set of relationship patterns in their interface with ECPs.

Father involvement in ECPs is defined as direct and indirect connections that fathers have with ECPs, including selecting programs, participating in program-related activities, assuming responsibility for children's health and wellbeing in the program, and supporting joint program and family goals. The research literature (e.g., Roggmann *et al.*, 2002; Goldman, 2005) strongly suggests that fathers who are highly involved with their young children are also more involved in ECPs. It is not the goal of this paper to examine the issues and literature related to father involvement in general, but rather to focus on involvement in ECPs and how to effectively encourage this type of involvement. The specific activities that are addressed as father involvement in ECPs include: communication with teachers, volunteering in the classroom, attending family events, participating in parenting education, home visits and program policy development.

The definitions and goals of ECPs are critical to understanding the literature about father involvement. In this paper, the following categories will be used as important categories for understanding ECP and their different goals. While early childhood has been defined as 0 to age 8 by the National Association for the Education of Young Children (NAEYC) (2008), the scope for this study will be more narrowly focused on programs for children ages 0–5. Childcare centers represent the largest group of ECPs and have the primary purpose of providing care for young children while parents are at work. There are a number of different programs that provide early education opportunities for young children who are at risk for poor educational outcomes. The Head Start and EHS Programs are national programs in the USA that have been serving this population of children for many years. A third type of ECP that serves young children with identified disabilities is Early Childhood Special Education which is home-based for 0- to 3-year olds and center based for 4- to 5-year-old children. Early Childhood Family Education is another ECP format where both parents and children attend a class together for the purpose of supporting the child's development toward school readiness through information and support for parents. The majority of research literature focuses on the first three types of programs with some limited practice literature on Early Childhood Family Education programs.

Ecological theory and fathers in ECPs

The ecological systems perspective refers to the adaptive fit between individuals and their environments. This perspective is particularly applicable for examining fathers and ECPs because of its focus on multiple system levels and the interrelationships among these systems. This perspective also provides a contextual view that fits with the current diversity of family systems and different types of ECPs. Bronfenbrenner and Morris (1998) suggest four levels of systems. The *microsystem* refers to the individual's immediate environments, such as the family or workplace. Fathers' participation in the ECP would constitute a microsystem influence on the family. *Exosystem* refers to the events that occur in immediate environments that do not directly involve the person. For example, staffing changes in the early childhood center may not directly involve the father but may have an indirect effect on him. The *mesosystem* entails the interaction of microsystems. For example, ECPs may impose holiday schedules that do not fit with the demands of fathers' work schedules. The intersection of these two systems may have an impact on the individual that goes beyond the influence of each individual system. *Macrosystem* refers to more remote influences on individuals such as social change and governmental policy. Bronfenbrenner (1986) suggests that individual behavior can best be understood within the context of this complex array of systems.

Most of the available research focuses on microsystem influences on fathers. Relevant microsystem influences may include family structure, parent attitudes about father involvement, parents' financial resources, and childcare policies and practices. Family structure has been shown to affect fathers' participation in ECPs. Qualitative research has suggested that nonresidential fathers may have difficulty staying involved in their child's ECP because mothers do not always communicate with them about events for parents (Fagan & Palm, 2004). However, survey research has not revealed significant differences between residential and nonresidential father involvement in Head Start as reported by mothers (Fagan et al., 2000), teachers, or objective assessments of the amount of time that fathers spend participating in their child's program (Fagan, 1999). Fatherhood demonstration programs in EHS have been shown to be more successful in efforts to involve resident fathers in programs compared with nonresident fathers (Raikes & Belotti, 2006). Given the inconclusive findings of these studies, we suggest that residence may be too broad a category for analysis. Researchers should begin to look more closely at the extent to which the association between residence and father involvement in ECPs is influenced by factors such as frequency of fathers' involvement with children at home or the quality of the mother–father relationship.

Attitudes about father involvement

Fathers' attitudes about their involvement in ECP activities also influence the degree to which they participate. The few available studies seem to suggest that, for the most part, fathers have positive attitudes about and interest in participating in ECPs. In a survey of 201 fathers with disabled children, 84% indicated that they probably would participate in activities designed for them (Hadadian & Merbler, 1995). In another study, fathers with children in one of four types of ECPs in six states: NAEYC-accredited childcare centers, Head Start programs, programs for infants and toddlers with disabilities, and programs for preschoolers with disabilities, were interviewed about their attitudes toward their involvement in their child's program (Turbiville *et al.*, 2000). Most fathers expressed interest in participating in their child's program, particularly in activities for the whole family. However, fathers with children in the NAEYC programs were mainly interested in 'Daddy and Me' groups, while fathers in Head Start programs expressed preferences for employment training and classroom volunteering.

Research has shown that mothers play a pivotal role in facilitating the father–child relationship in the environment of the home (Walker & McGraw, 2000). Mothers may also encourage or discourage fathers from participating in ECPs either directly or indirectly. For example, mothers may arrange their work schedules so they are more available to drop off or pick up their children from the program, thus, discouraging fathers from being involved in their children's program. Few research studies have actually examined mothers' attitudes and role in facilitating father involvement in ECPs. A study of 59 low-income Head Start families living in urban, suburban and rural settings showed that while fathers were perceived to be either quite or very involved with their children at home, they were not very involved in Head Start (Fagan *et al.*, 2000). However, mothers were satisfied with fathers' low involvement in Head Start, suggesting that mothers did not perceive fathers' lack of involvement as an issue. This low level of father involvement in Head Start may be related to the lack of encouragement from mothers.

The few existing studies suggest that some teachers and mothers are not especially eager to involve fathers in ECPs (McBride & Rane, 2001). Therefore, one challenge to researchers will be to determine the degree to which changing teachers' and mothers' attitudes may make a difference in the involvement of fathers in ECPs. Research is also needed to gain a better understanding of the ways in which fatherhood program initiatives affect change in attitudes about father involvement. Father involvement in early childhood settings is still a relatively new phenomenon. Considering the fact that mothers have for the most part dominated in this arena, it seems logical to assume that fathers will need to be supported by all adults, including mothers and teachers, if their level of involvement is to increase.

Another microsystem variable that may influence father involvement in ECPs is men's parenting behavior and style. Research has shown that authoritative parents tend to spend more time directly engaged with their children at home than authoritarian parents. Fathers who reported higher levels of nurturance toward their children also spent more total time in their child's Head Start program (Fagan, 1999). Fathers also tend to become more involved in their child's Head Start program when they are better educated, less depressed and more likely to use social support (Roggman *et al.*, 2002).

Patterns and levels of father involvement in ECPs

Studies of fathers' involvement in ECPs have examined participation in home visitation sessions, group activities for children and group activities for parents, drop-off and pick-up, communication with teachers and care givers, and assumption of responsibility for childcare. The small number of surveys conducted on father involvement in ECPs reveals low levels of father participation. One of the first father involvement surveys was conducted in a Head Start program in Washington, DC (Gary *et al.*, 1987). Three-fourths of the 118 fathers in the study reported that they participated in Head Start activities only a few times per year or not at all. Similarly, a large, pre-kindergarten 'at risk' program in Illinois found that father participation in parent activities accounted for less than 5% of the total parent participation (McBride & Lin, 1996). At the time that the data were collected, however, the program had done little to reach out to fathers of children in the program. When a formal fatherhood initiative is implemented, fathers' participation in program activities increases significantly (Raikes & Belotti, 2006). For example, a Head Start initiative emphasising fathers' classroom volunteering revealed that about twice as many intervention group fathers were involved in the classroom as control group fathers (52% versus 27%) over the course of the school year (Fagan, 1999).

Qualitative research with fathers in different types of ECPs revealed that Head Start fathers' participation differed in quantity and quality from fathers in other types of ECPs (Fagan & Palm, 2004). Head Start fathers who became actively involved in the program appeared to value their participation for its generative contribution to their children and the wider community. This attitude was reflected not only in the fathers' ideas about changing negative perceptions of fathers in the community and helping other men who are having difficulty with family relationships, but also in fathers' commitment to support and form bonds with other children in the program who seemed to need such relationships. There was no instance in the other ECPs where fathers became involved with other people's children.

Researchers should continue to focus on patterns and levels of father involvement in ECPs. In addition, there is little consensus among researchers about methods for measuring fathers' involvement in ECPs. Most studies have focused on levels of participation, such as amount of time volunteering in the classroom or number of classroom visits. Researchers need to develop valid and reliable measures of program involvement. Further, few studies have examined the quality of fathers' involvement. The child development literature alerts us to the importance of assessing the quality and quantity of father involvement with children in the home environment. We can only assume that measures of quality may be as or more important than measures of quantity of involvement in ECPs.

Program variables

The ecological perspective suggests that programmatic variables are likely to impact fathers' participation in the ECP. One such variable is the type of ECP. Very little research has been conducted with fathers that have children in day care centers or family day care programs. A small-scale day care center study revealed that middle-income fathers are just as likely as mothers to drop their children off at the center, but men are less likely to pick up the child, presumably because fathers tend to work longer hours at their jobs than mothers (Fagan, 1997). Fathers engaged in many of the same activities in the center as mothers, although they were significantly less likely than mothers to communicate with day care staff members (Fagan, 1997).

Evolution of an agency's fatherhood initiative is an exosystem variable in the sense that the program changes do not directly involve the father but may have an indirect effect on him. McAllister *et al.* (2004) identified five stages of program maturation. In Stage 1, the roles and needs of fathers were sometimes discussed with mothers, but the mother–child dyad was the main focus of the program. In Stage 2, the program made efforts to involve fathers, but primarily through male-only activities. In Stage 3, there was a shift from male-only activities for fathers to including fathers in all aspects of the program, including home visits, family goal planning, intake, etc. In Stage 4, the program staff began to think more holistically about fathers. Staff engaged fathers in relation to their parenting concerns, but they also worked with men around their own personal goals. In Stage 5, fathers are viewed as co-parents. Staff also think more reflectively about the father's relationship to his child, and they encourage fathers and mother to think reflectively about their own relationships to the child.

This type of research has the potential to help practitioners think more critically about the development of their programs and to set goals that they had not previously considered. For example, practitioners may be focused only on how to involve as many fathers as possible or how to implement good quality programs. They may not be thinking about ways to move the program toward increasingly complex programming.

Future research should focus on several important research questions pertaining to program development. How do programs at various stages of maturity affect fathers' engagement with children? How do the stages of fatherhood program development affect other aspects of ECPs, including staff retention and job satisfaction?

Mesosystem and macrosystem variables

Very few studies have examined mesosystem influences on father involvement in ECPs. One such study examined the relationship between fathers workplace supports and their participation in their child's ECP—fathers were more engaged in their child's program when they had flexible employers, defined as allowing employees to bring work home on occasion, take time off to care for sick children, and to attend school events (Fagan & Press, 2008). Further, mothers reported higher levels of work–family balance when fathers had flexible jobs and when fathers assumed greater responsibility for childcare (Fagan & Press). There is clearly a need for more research examining mesosystem influences on fathers. For example, to what extent do fathers become involved in ECPs when employers provide time to fathers to attend school meetings and conferences during work hours.

We are not aware of research examining macrosystem influences on fathers and ECPs. Research is needed to examine whether day care quality improvement initiatives at the State and Federal levels in the USA have resulted in more positive partnerships between fathers (or mothers) and ECPs. We are not aware of any research that has examined the effects of State childcare subsidies on fathers' involvement in their child's ECP. Subsidies may enable fathers to take extra time from work (i.e., reduce the need to work overtime) to spend in their child's program.

Situated fathering and ECPs

Situated fathering (Marsiglio *et al.*, 2005) provides a different lens for understanding father involvement in ECPs. The focus is on the ECPs as unique microsystems. The physical, social and symbolic characteristics of ECPs are complementary dimensions of the more general ecological perspective that was presented in the last section. The exploration of the physical and social characteristics expands our understanding of the microsystem environments of ECPs. This section will incorporate both empirical research on ECPs as well as the 'practice literature' on developing fatherhood programs as applied to early childhood settings. Situated fathering as a conceptual framework has identified the following set of primary characteristics: physical properties, temporal dynamics, symbolic, social structure and public/private spaces. In addition, a secondary set of characteristics, institutional/cultural, transitional, personal power and control, gendered attributes and fatherhood discourses are also proposed as important aspects of understanding fatherhood under various circumstances. The situated fathering framework has been used to explore a number of different situations including fathers in prison, fathers in the military, long haul truck drivers and responsible fatherhood programs (Marsiglio *et al.*, 2005). The situations that were analysed with the situated fathering model were generally 'masculine' environments while ECPs would typically be identified as 'feminine' environments.

Primary characteristics

Physical properties.   Early childhood settings are child-centered—they have child-sized furniture and a variety of play and educational materials arranged into different interest areas. These may be literacy centers with books and writing materials, dramatic play area with dress up clothes, dolls and other props for play. These areas typically reflect home activities that might be associated with stay at home parents (mothers). There may also be areas for art activities, tables for eating and small motor activities, and a block area with trains, cars, trucks and other vehicles. The colors and décor in rooms often reflect feminine preferences since most staff members in programs are women. Programs may also have gyms, large muscle areas and outdoor play areas that may feel more comfortable and familiar to men than the typical classroom. Burgess and

Bartlett (2005) suggest that the 'décor is not overtly "feminine"-colours (pink) and borders (not flowers)' (p. 16). They also suggest a toilet area marked for men, children's books about fathers and children, and male-icon toys like cars and action men. While most early childhood spaces include some areas or materials that may be more familiar to fathers they often reflect a feminine bias in how they are decorated, equipped and arranged. The practice literature has provided some direction for creating father-friendly physical environments (e.g., Levine *et al.*, 1993; Fagan & Palm, 2004; Burgess & Bartlett, 2005).

Temporal dynamics. The literature mentions time constraints that many fathers face in relationship with being involved in ECPs (Johnson & Palm, 1992). For many fathers, daytime hours of programs or program activities such as volunteering or going on field trips do not fit with their work schedules. This is especially true for men with less flexible jobs. The practice literature has suggested that evening and weekend hours are more likely to be accessible to fathers (Fagan & Palm, 2004). McBride (1990) and Palm (1998) describe programs for fathers and their young children that met on Saturday mornings in early childhood settings.

Symbolic. Fathers will come to early childhood settings with some preconceived ideas about the program. They may connect them with the more formal educational settings, which may have some negative connotations depending upon their own experiences with schools (Fletcher & Daly, 2002; Goldman, 2005). Some ECPs are more formal and structured and more closely reflect the educational institutions while others can be less formal and emphasise child play as the primary pathway to learning. Men may resonate more with the less formal settings that emphasise play. When the dramatic play areas focus more on female familiar activities such as housekeeping and doll play, fathers may feel out of their comfort zones. Palm (1992) suggests using more male-oriented play themes and props as one way to make fathers feel more comfortable engaging in dramatic play activities. Programs that use a gym or large motor environment may find that this appeals to men who have more familiarity and comfort with the activities that take place in this type of environment. It is still necessary for programs to guide fathers into activities that are appropriate for young children in these environments. A gym with basketball hoops will attract men to shoot baskets, but this activity is not appropriate for young children under five.

Social structure. The social structure of the early childhood environment typically includes teachers who are predominately if not exclusively female. The staff members have power over the programs in that they design the environment and set the rules and norms for the environment. Fathers may be given some privileges related to their guest status in this environment, but this also sends the message that their presence is unusual and not expected on a regular basis. One of the authors has experienced this sentiment in observations of fathers who attend family education programs.

Teachers can be too welcoming and give fathers a special status in the program, which would not be given to mothers. The social structure in programs like Head Start may also include decision-making bodies like the Policy Council where fathers experience male privilege (Fagan & Palm, 2004). This type of social structure does not reflect gender equity and may define specific roles and expectations for fathers that limit areas and levels of involvement while at the same time giving fathers a privileged position when they do choose to become involved. Males who are involved in female-dominated social institutions like ECPs enter situations where they are not expected and then are often treated as privileged guests.

Public/private spaces.   The typical early childhood environment is a public space and is shared with both children from other families and adults (teachers and other parents). The public nature of this space may make it less comfortable for some fathers where parenting in public may feel threatening especially with other adults who may judge one's parenting. It is interesting to note that fathers are most interested in participating in family activities in ECPs (e.g., Palm, 1985; Turbiville *et al.*, 2000). It may be that fathers feel more secure coming as a family than as a lone parent. Fagan (1999) reports that fathers are more likely to be involved in ECPs when mothers are involved in the program. Being with their family makes this a more private space for fathers and buffers them in the presence of others. The research literature (Raikes *et al.*, 2005) also reports that home visitation is associated with increased father participation. There may be two factors at work here. First is the comfort of being in one's home and second is the convenience of having someone come to you. Fathers are more comfortable in their own homes and this may be the best place to initiate father involvement in early education. Raikes *et al.* (2005) point out that home visits may be a mechanism for reaching non-English speaking and less educated fathers.

Secondary characteristics

Gendered attributes.   Goldman (2005) describes schools as feminised institutions and this same case could be made for early childhood settings. The vast majority of teachers/staff were female (96%) in preprimary settings in 25 countries (OECD, 2007). This influences the physical environment as described above and also shapes the activities in ECPs. The importance of gender of staff in relation to recruiting father involvement in programs is documented in EHS research (Raikes *et al.*, 2005) where programs that were more mature had higher levels of father involvement. Mature programs typically had experienced male staff members. Burgess and Bartlett (2005) provide a list of suggestions for creating a 'male presence' in programs as a way to address the predominance of female staff. The discussion of male versus female staff for fatherhood programs continues to be an issue (Bartlett & Vann, 2004; MFFN, 2007). Some programs have made efforts to recruit male staff as one way to address this gender imbalance.

Activities also can reflect the feminisation in ECPs. The dramatic play areas and activities may reflect a more feminine bias with the typical housekeeping area or beauty shop versus a car repair or camping set of props. Circle time songs and finger plays may also be unfamiliar and uncomfortable for some men (Palm, 1997). The influence of staff gender on activities has not been explored in a systematic manner in early childhood settings.

Fatherhood discourses. Different ECPs have different goals and different target populations which reflect different discourses and father involvement opportunities. Head Start programs for male involvement have been created to address father absence and support father responsibility (Turbiville *et al.*, 2000). The history of Head Start as part of the War on Poverty led to the focus on parent empowerment and parent involvement through volunteer work and decision-making. The research on father involvement in Head Start and EHS suggests that men of color are involved in these programs at a higher level than white fathers (Raikes *et al.*, 2005). These fathers are interested in supporting their child's success in school. Fagan and Palm (2004) also found that African-American fathers express a strong commitment to the larger community as male role models for children. The differences in participation by race raise interesting questions about different goals for father involvement. Fathers in Head Start were involved as both volunteers and as members of the Policy Council, which fit with both the goals of the programs and the discourses around fatherhood for these programs where father absence has been stressed as detrimental to young children. Fathers are involved to help their child succeed in school and may also feel an obligation to address this issue of father absence in African-American communities.

The goal for childcare programs is to provide parents with care and education for children while parents are working. The discourse related to fatherhood is that both mothers and fathers are sharing the provider role and responsibility for childcare and household tasks. Parent involvement in childcare programs includes dropping children off and picking them up. Fathers with children in childcare programs in the Fagan and Palm (2004) study expressed reluctance to engage in other types of involvement that might limit the amount of time they had to spend with their child at home. While the discourse around increasing father involvement in ECPs is important to professionals, fathers may perceive that their involvement beyond dropping off or picking up a child is in conflict with their work roles. They are in effect sub-contracting to childcare programs the care of their children while they are at work so that they can work and provide for their family. Their level of involvement with their children at home may not spill over into the childcare setting the way it does when their children begin school in the K-12 system. While many families use childcare services and it is an important connection to fathers, fathers' attitudes toward parenting involvement options such as volunteering and parent education need to be studied in more depth.

Early education/school readiness programs focus on children getting ready for school. Fathers' role in getting children ready for school can be addressed by fathers supporting early literacy at home (e.g., reading to young children). There may be other opportunities for parent involvement in family events or home visits that might appeal to fathers and support their role as teachers and supporters of their children's education. The discourse here is around father's role and his perception of his role as a teacher (Ortiz et al., 1999). As ECP discourse is more focused on early education and preparation for school, fathers' attitudes toward involvement may change.

Early intervention programs for young children with disabilities focus on supporting children's development. Programs can involve fathers by helping them to understand and accept their child's disability and serve as a support person for their partner. Fathers may be involved in parent education programs, home visits and conferences in this type of ECP. The discourse about fatherhood is how to engage fathers in understanding and accepting their child's disability and the implications for future development. Some fathers may approach this as a problem to solve and overcome (Pelchat et al., 2007) and become strong advocates for their child.

Early Childhood Family Education programs focus on improving parent knowledge, skill and support. The discourse about fatherhood is focused on the goal of creating warm, close and supportive relationships with young children. Parent education is the primary focus and strategy in this type of program (Palm, 1998). This type of program often includes parent–child play time (e.g., McBride, 1990; Palm, 1992) that provides fathers with a space for undistracted 'quality time' with their child as well as opportunities to learn from observing and talking with other fathers.

The opportunities for father involvement vary for different programs, as do the goals of each program. This clearly impacts the kind of discourse about fatherhood that occurs for each program and the types of involvement opportunities that may appeal to fathers. ECPs have demonstrated different levels of involvement (Turbiville et al., 2000). This analysis about goals and the discourse about father involvement help to explain the differences as related to these situational factors.

Summary of situated fathering analysis

This analysis reflects the diversity of ECPs and the different goals and involvement activities that might be used to engage fathers. Increasing positive father involvement is a shared goal across settings but takes on different meanings for fathers depending on the program goals, race/culture of fathers and father's perception of the child's needs. Father-only activities may be one way to create a 'male space' within an ECP that supports men in exploring their roles and learning new information and skills. The father's level of involvement with their child is an important factor in how involved they may be in ECPs, but it is mediated by their perceptions of the goals of the program and the involvement opportunities that programs make accessible to fathers.

Studies of the impact of fatherhood programs on fathers and children

The ecological and situated fathering perspectives address various issues regarding the intersection between fathers, families and ECPS, but they say little about the impact of father involvement in ECPs on fathers and children. A small number of outcome studies using varying degrees of research rigor have been published to date. Studies that examined father participation in multiple program activities have shown positive effects on some aspects of fathering and child outcomes. For example, Fagan and Iglesias (1999) explored the effects of Head Start fathers' participation in a program that included three components: classroom volunteering, attendance at organised fun activities and a monthly support group. Fathers in the intervention group showed significantly greater gains in direct interaction and support for learning activities with children at home than the comparison group of fathers, but only if the fathers were at least moderately involved in the program. Also, children of high involvement, intervention group fathers showed greater gains in mathematics readiness than children of low involvement, comparison group fathers. In another study, fathers with children enrolled in EHS employed significantly more complex social play interactions with their 24-month olds than did fathers with children in the control group (no EHS services) (Roggman *et al.*, 2004). The largest study to date is the EHS study, which includes fathers in 17 demonstration sites and a control group. Results of the this study revealed that fathers in the EHS program spanked children less, and children engaged their fathers in more play, compared with control families (ACF, 2002).

Positive effects in fathering were also found in a study that assessed the impact of one program component. Fagan and Stevenson (2002) evaluated the effect of an empowerment-based parent education program for Head Start fathers in which they were trained to lead the structured self-help program on fathering. For the experimental group, there was a significant improvement in fathers' attitudes about their ability to teach their children. Also, resident fathers in the experimental group showed significant gains in self-esteem and parenting satisfaction.

Summary and implications for research and practice

Father involvement in ECPs has been explored as an important microsystem context for encouraging positive father–child relationships that will benefit the development of young children. This review of current research and practice literature begins to identify factors that support increased father involvement in ECPs as well as barriers to father involvement. Fathers' characteristics (residence, mental health, education, race, parenting style, attitudes about involvement and beliefs about program involvement) are identified as influencing the level of involvement. Family factors (mothers' attitudes, mothers' employment, mother–father relationships) are also related to fathers' level of involvement. Program characteristics (teacher attitudes, program goals, parent involvement opportunities, program maturity in relationship to father involvement) also appear to be important in mediating the level of father involvement. More systematic research of father involvement in ECPs has to begin with a consistent definition of father involvement that assesses both quantity and quality of involvement.

ECPs include a diverse set of programs and services that represent different goals for families and children. The role of father involvement in these different program contexts has not been studied in a way that differentiates program goals and beliefs about father involvement. It has been assumed that increased father involvement in ECPs is an important and realistic goal for all programs. This review suggests that ECPs represent a diverse array of goals and strategies for father involvement that reflect different program purposes and family and community contexts. Recruitment of fathers is a common challenge among programs but opportunities for father involvement should be consistent with the primary goals of programs. Creating father-friendly ECPs requires an understanding of the needs of fathers and families in specific community contexts and designing appropriate and meaningful opportunities for father involvement that are consistent with program goals.

Outcome studies of fatherhood program initiatives are sorely lacking. The field should make every effort to encourage more research on outcomes for fathers, children and families. These studies are challenging to implement but necessary for providing evidence of the effects of fatherhood programs. Future outcome studies should include measures of dosage and intensity of involvement in the program as well as examine the impacts of different types of program involvement (e.g., classroom volunteering, attendance at support groups). Research also needs to address the extent to which programs are successful at affecting different sub-groups of fathers (e.g., resident versus nonresident fathers) and the extent to which fatherhood programs impact children.

References

ACF (Administration for Children, Youth, and Families). (2002) *Making a difference in the lives of infants and toddlers and their families* (Washington, DC, Department of Health and Human Services).

Bartlett, D. & Vann, N. (2004) Review of the state of practical work, in: D. Lemieux (Ed) *Supporting fathers: contributions from the international fatherhood summit 2003* (The Hague, Bernard van Leer Foundation), 78–107.

Bronfenbrenner, U. (1986) Ecology of the family as a context for human development: research perspectives, *Developmental Psychology*, 22, 723–742.

Bronfenbrenner, U. & Morris, P. A. (1998) The ecology of developmental processes, in: W. Damon & R. M. Lerner (Eds) *Handbook of child psychology: theoretical models of human development* (Vol. 1, 5th edn) (Hoboken, NJ, John Wiley), 993–1028.

Burgess, A. & Bartlett, D. (2005) *Working with fathers: a guide for everyone working with families* (London, Fathers Direct).

Cabrera, N. (2004) Guest editorial, *Fathering: A Journal of Theory, Research, and Practice about Men as Fathers*, 2(1), 1–4.

Fagan, J. (1997) Patterns of mother and father involvement in child care, *Child and Youth Care Forum*, 26, 113–126.

Fagan, J. (1999) *Predictors of father and father figure involvement in pre-kindergarten Head Start* (Philadelphia, PA, National Center on Fathers and Families).

Fagan, J. & Iglesias, A. (1999) Father and father figure involvement in Head Start: a quasi-experimental study, *Early Childhood Research Quarterly*, 14, 243–269.

Fagan, J., Newash, N. & Scholesser, A. (2000) Female caregivers' perceptions of fathers' and significant adult males' involvement with their Head Start children, *Families in Society*, 81, 186–196.

Fagan, J. & Palm, G. (2004) *Fathers and early childhood programs* (Clifton Heights, NY, Delmar).

Fagan, J. & Press, J. (2008) Father influences on employed mothers' work-family balance, *Journal of Family Issues*, 29, 1136–1160.

Fagan, J. & Stevenson, H. (2002) An experimental study of an empowerment-based intervention for African American Head Start fathers, *Family Relations*, 51, 191–198.

Fletcher, R. & Daly, K. (2002) *Fathers' involvement in their children's literacy development* (Newcastle, Family Action Center, University of Newcastle).

Gary, L., Beatty, L. & Weaver, G. (1987) *Involvement of black fathers in Head Start.* Report submitted to the Department of Health and Human Services, ACYF, Grant No. 90-CD-0509 (Washington, DC, Institute for Urban Affairs and Research, Howard University).

Goldman, R. (2005) *Fathers' involvement in their children's education* (London, National Family and Parenting Institute).

Hadadian, A. & Merbler, J. (1995) Fathers of young children with disabilities: how do they want to be involved? *Child and Youth Care Forum*, 24, 327–338.

Johnson, L. & Palm, G. (1992) Planning programs: what do fathers want? in: L. Johnson & G. Palm (Eds) *Working with fathers: methods and perspectives* (Stillwater, MN, nu ink), 59–77.

Levine, J., Murphy, D. & Wilson, S. (1993) *Getting men involved: strategies for early childhood programs* (New York, Scholastic).

Lewis, C. & Lamb, M. (2004) Fathers: the research perspective, in: D. Lemieux (Ed) *Supporting fathers: contributions from the international fatherhood summit 2003* (The Hague, Bernard van Leer Foundation), 45–77.

Marsiglio, W., Roy, K. & Fox, G. L. (Eds) (2005) *Situated fathering: a focus on physical and social spaces* (Lanham, MD, Rowman & Littlefield).

McAllister, C. L., Wilson, P. C. & Burton, J. (2004) From sports fans to nurturers: an EHS program's evolution toward father involvement, *Fathering: A Journal of Theory, Research, and Practice about Men as Fathers*, 2, 31–59.

McBride, B. A. (1990) The effects of parent education/play group program on father involvement in child rearing, *Family Relations*, 39, 250–256.

McBride, B. A. & Lin, H. F. (1996) Parental involvement in pre-kindergarten at-risk programs: multiple perspectives, *Journal of Education for Students Placed at Risk*, 1, 349–372.

McBride, B. A. & Lutz, M. M. (2004) Intervention: changing the nature and extent of father involvement, in: M. Lamb (Ed.) *The role of the father in child development* (4th edn) (Hoboken, NJ, John Wiley), 446–475.

McBride, B. A. & Rane, T. R. (2001) Father/male involvement in early childhood programs: training staff to work with men, in: J. Fagan & A. J. Hawkins (Eds) *Clinical and education interventions with fathers* (Binghamton, NY, Haworth), 171–190.

McLanahan, S. & Carlson, M. S. (2004) Fathers in fragile families, in: M. Lamb (Ed.) *The role of the father in child development* (4th edn) (Hoboken, NJ, John Wiley), 368–396.

Minnesota Fathers & Families Network (MFFN) (2007) *Do we count father: searching for key indicators of well-being of fathers and families* (St. Paul, MN, Author).

National Association for the Education of Young Children (2008) Available online at: http://www.naeyc.org/about

OECD (Organisation for Economic Co-operation and Development). (2007) *Education at a Glance 2007: OECD Indicators* (Paris, Organisation for Economic Co-operation and Development).

Ortiz, R., Stile, S. & Brown, C. (1999) Early literacy activities of fathers: reading and writing with young children, *Young Children*, 55(5), 16–18.

Palm, G. (1985) Creating opportunities for father involvement, *Nurturing News*, 7(4), 4, 11–12.

Palm, G. (1992) Building intimacy and parenting skills through father–child activity time, in: L. Johnson & G. Palm (Eds) *Working with fathers: methods and perspectives* (Stillwater, MN, nu ink), 79–100.

Palm, G. (1997) Promoting generative fathering through parent and family education, in: A. J. Hawkins & D. C. Dollahite (Eds) *Generative fathering: beyond deficit perspectives* (Thousand Oaks, CA, Sage), 167–182.

Palm, G. (1998) *Super Saturdays: lessons from a program for dads and kids* (St. Cloud, MN, District 742 Community Education).

Pelchat, D., Lefebvre, H. & Levert, M. (2007) Gender differences and similarities in the experience of parenting a child with a health problem: current state of knowledge, *Journal of Health Care*, 11(2), 112–131.

Pruett, K. (2000) *Fatherneed: why father care is as essential as mother care for your child* (New York, Free Press).

Raikes, H. & Belotti, J. (2006) Two studies of father involvement in Early Head Start Programs: a national survey and a demonstration program evaluation, *Parenting: Science and Practice*, 6, 229–242.

Raikes, H. H., Summers, J. A. & Roggmann, L. A. (2005) Fathering involvement in EHS programs, *Fathering: A Journal of Theory, Research, and Practice about Men as Fathers*, 3, 29–58.

Roggmann, L. A., Boyce, L. K., Cook, G. A. & Cook, J. (2002) Getting dads involved: predictors of father involvement in Early Head Start and with their children, *Infant Mental Health Journal*, 23, 62–78.

Roggman, L. A., Boyce, L. K., Cook, G. A., Christiansen, K. & Jones, D. (2004) Playing with daddy: social toy play, early head start and developmental outcomes. *Fathering: A Journal of Theory, Research, and Practice about Men as Fathers*, 2, 83–108.

Turbiville, V. P., Umbarger, G. T. & Guthrie, A. C. (2000) Fathers' involvement in programs for young children, *Young Children*, 55, 74–79.

Walker, A. J. & McGraw, L. A. (2000) Who is responsible for responsible fathering? *Journal of Marriage and the Family*, 62, 563–569.

'Something in it for dads': getting fathers involved with Sure Start

Carol Potter[a] and John Carpenter[b]

[a]Carnegie Faculty of Sport and Education, Leeds Metropolitan University, UK; [b]School for Policy Studies, University of Bristol, UK

Introduction

The Labour government's green paper *Every child matters* (DfES, 2003) stated, 'We should recognise the vital role played by fathers as well as mothers' (p. 20). Reviewing 21 research studies related to fathers in the UK, Lewis (2000) concluded that 'the current policy interest in fathers is the culmination of three decades of rapid change in the institutions and conventions of family life' (p. 2).

There is substantial evidence that when fathers are more involved with caring for their children, then children often do better in later life, particularly in their psychological and social development (e.g. Lamb, 2004). Head Start researchers in the USA found that where fathers had been highly involved, children did better in school and where less so, children tended to show more behavioural problems (Fagan & Iglesias, 1999). Dubowitz *et al.* (2001) found that the presence of a father in families of six year olds was associated not only with increased cognitive development but also with a sense of greater competence by the children themselves.

Despite these known benefits of fathers' involvement, it has been generally acknowledged that the practice of providing effective support to fathers in their parenting role continues to lag far behind policy aspirations (Lewis, 2000; O'Brien, 2004). The National Family and Parenting Institute's mapping of family services in England and Wales (Henricson *et al.*, 2001) recorded that fewer than 1% of family services were targeted at fathers and that fathers 'are not perceived to be in the mainstream of provision and face barriers to support' (p. 7). In their review of family centres, Ghate *et al.* (2000) concluded that:

> Provision of services for men as child carers lags behind that for women. Fathers are neither well served by family support services nor are they widely catered for in their own right. (Ghate *et al.*, 2000, p. 2)

There are a number of widely acknowledged structural and attitudinal reasons for low father engagement in family services, a full discussion of which is beyond the scope of this paper. However, major factors include the following: father perceptions that such services are 'for mothers' and there being significant justification for such a perception (Ghate *et al.*, 2000); traditional belief systems which see fathers as economic providers and mothers as childcarers (Goldman, 2005); professional reluctance to engage men (Ryan, 2000) and male reluctance to seek help and advice (Lloyd, 2001).

Sure Start

The introduction of Sure Start, a major New Labour initiative aimed at alleviating disadvantage in the early years, was intended to achieve change in the area of father involvement with early guidance documents exhorting local programmes to include parents in all aspects of the planning, managing and running of services. They were required to 'Involve parents, grandparents and other carers in ways that build on their existing strengths' (DfEE, 1999). The strong inference was that programmes should adopt a broad service delivery approach, which included fathers. However, Lloyd *et al.* (2003) found that 36% of 118 round 1 and 2 programmes gave only a low priority to working with fathers, 52% a medium one and only 12% had made it a high priority in their work. More recently, a report produced by the National Evaluation of Sure Start, reviewing developments within the programmes during their first four years spoke of a 'low overall level of father involvement in programmes' (Tunstill *et al.*, 2005). Such findings demonstrate that despite explicit guidance that local Sure

Start programmes should seek to involve fathers, only a minority apparently sought to do so in a comprehensive fashion. Sure Start Hinton, the subject of this study, was one such programme.

Research aim

The aim of this study was to find out to what extent fathers were engaged with Sure Start Hinton and to determine which strategies fathers, mothers and programme staff believed to be most effective in engaging men. Father and mother perceptions of the many benefits of engagement with the programme are discussed elsewhere in this paper.

Research design

The case study presented concerns a Sure Start local programme in the north east of England. Sure Start Hinton was established in 2000 and became operational in 2001. Specific services for fathers and male carers began to be set up in 2002.

This study took place in the context of a five-year independent evaluation of a number of programmes in the area. Where possible, and with the agreement of the Programme Partnership Boards, evaluations were linked in order to make relevant comparisons of process and outcomes. For this study, the comparator programme operated within the same county as Sure Start Hinton and provided information about its activities for fathers and data on their involvement. This comparator programme would best be described in terms of Lloyd *et al.*'s (2003) criteria as giving 'medium priority' to fathers.

The impact of Sure Start Hinton's work is assessed quantitatively, comparing the two programmes in terms of the numbers of fathers engaged and the total number of attendances per year. Engagement and attendance data were collated for the years 2002–2005 from the programmes' databases. The collection of such data is a requirement of funding and both programmes used the same software and methods. Perspectives on the nature of strategies perceived to be effective in engaging men are then discussed in relation to the views of fathers, mothers and Sure Start Hinton staff.

In order to obtain parents' views, a convenience sample of 16 fathers and one grandfather with care of the children was recruited and eight mothers, partners of some of these men, also agreed to take part. Fifteen fathers were married; 11 of these were employed and the other four were unemployed and had full-time care of their children. The other two were unmarried, unemployed and had sole care of the children.

Semi-structured interviews were undertaken with nine of the fathers and the eight mothers. Twelve fathers participated in four focus groups organised on the basis of attendance at particular programme activities such as a Childcare course and a 'Dads Drop in' session.

Staff perspectives were obtained from semi-structured interviews with three members of Sure Start Hinton staff, namely the Fathers Worker, the Programme

Manager and the Health Visitor Co-ordinator and with the director of an expert voluntary organisation working with fathers in the north east of England.

Data analysis

All focus group and interview data were transcribed and a summary of each returned to each participant as a mechanism for checking the trustworthiness of the data (Robson, 2002). Data analysis was undertaken using NVIVO qualitative software program. A grounded theory approach was adopted (Strauss & Corbin, 1990) where the development of theory is inductively derived from the study of the phenomenon which it represents. Specifically, data analysis took place in three stages. Initially, first level general thematic categories were identified, following which, a number of sub themes within each of these wider categories emerged. Finally, direct quotations representing each sub theme were selected to provide a rich description of the perceptions of fathers and mothers.

Findings

Fathers' engagement and attendance

The number of fathers engaged in the Hinton programme's activities increased from three in 2002 to over a hundred in 2005. This compares to an average of 7.5 fathers in the comparator programme (Figure 1).

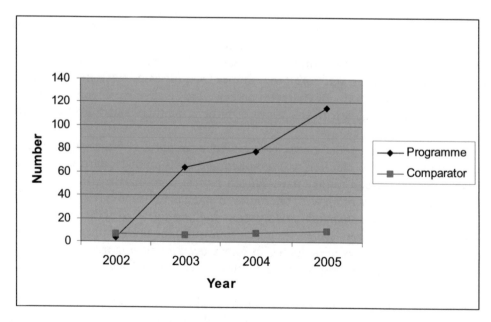

Figure 1.   Fathers engaged in programme

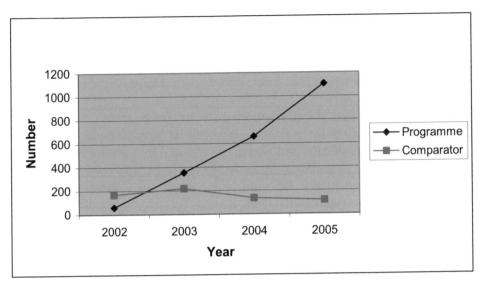

Figure 2. Total attendances

The total number of male attendances at Sure Start Hinton's activities rose from 60 to over 1000 in 2005, whereas in the comparator programme it started higher but declined in the last two years (Figure 2).

The men were involved at all levels of the Hinton Sure Start programme, from attendance at a range of activities through to membership of the Parents' Group and Sure Start Partnership, the governing body of Sure Start programmes. However, it is important to note that over 90% of all attendances after 2003 were recorded at male-specific activities and events.

Getting fathers/male carers involved: what worked

We now explore the reasons for Sure Start Hinton's apparent success in engaging large numbers of fathers and male carers. Factors at both strategic and everyday levels can be shown to have been important in the creation of a whole systems approach to working with men.

Strategic level

The programme's early and continuing commitment to active involvement for men appears to have been especially important. Despite a slow start to the programme's work in this area, witnessed by the regular involvement of only three fathers in 2002, programme managers continued to support fathers' work strongly over a number of years.

The second strategic factor perceived to contribute significantly to programme success in engaging fathers was a close working relationship with a local voluntary organisation having expertise in the process of male engagement. The programme manager believed that staff input from this agency was of 'fundamental' importance in developing the work with fathers and male carers. The voluntary agency supported the appointment and training of a part-time Fathers Worker and entered into a successful dual management of this member of staff. The agency also delivered extensive staff training to the whole Sure Start team since the launch of programme services in 2001.

A third factor identified at a strategic level was the programme's consistent use of a gender differentiated approach which sets out to recognise and address the different needs and interests of men and women as opposed to a gender blind approach, which treats men and women in approximately the same way (Ghate *et al.*, 2000). Providing all-male activities is one important aspect of a gender differentiated approach, as is the introduction of a dedicated worker to focus specifically on involving fathers.

Programme delivery level

Skills and abilities of the dedicated Fathers Worker

At the everyday level of programme working, both staff and fathers/male carers considered that the skills of the Fathers Worker were fundamental in engaging men locally. In general, men felt strongly that the worker was doing a very good job:

> She is an excellent worker. (F (father) 6)

> She does a really cracking job. (F15)

In particular, staff and fathers/male carers emphasised the importance of the worker's persistence:

> Persuading people—she's never heard the word 'no'. (F12)

Hard work and positive outlook were also valued by fathers and male carers:

> She's just so enthusiastic—to me—it's partly her enthusiasm I think—I wish I was as enthusiastic in my job. (F4)

The female Fathers Worker's ability to relate well to men was highlighted:

> She just joins in—she's like one of the lads—she supports you and she even joins in—you know you could get other people and you could be uncomfortable type—whereas [the Fathers Worker] just goes along with it. (F13)

The importance of humour in all-male groups was emphasised by a number of fathers and male carers. One father said:

> Men Mickey take all the time—specially when you get a group of men together—you've got to have banter—if you haven't got banter you haven't got a group. (F6)

Finally, the use of an individualised approach was valued:

> She doesn't treat you like a number—she treats you like an individual person. (F2)

A social marketing approach

Another key factor was the implicit use of an assertive social marketing approach where activities and events are 'sold' to fathers and male carers on the basis of explaining what they and their families can gain from them (McDermott, 2000).

The worker herself stated:

> There's got to be something in it for dads or they're not going to do it—at the end of the day, the programme has to ask 'why would fathers choose to come in?'

There are three critical stages in the approach: First, the worker, in close collaboration with her two line managers, set out to identify the most attractive 'products' through a process of explicit consultation with fathers and male carers. Several fathers commented on the importance of this strategy:

> [the dads worker] keeps on saying 'what do you want to do?'—she's always asking that—or trips wise—is there anywhere that we want to go? And if the funding's there we can get something sorted. (F1)

The second stage is to act on the suggestions quickly and consistently, so that there is a variety of activities being developed at any given time to maintain interest. The final and most critical stage is 'selling' the activities to individuals. The worker concerned seemed particularly adept at doing this, as one remarked:

> The way she does it is excellent—she'll come up to you and say 'this class will be very good for you—would you like to do it? We can sort out funding, I'll help you with this and I'll help you with that' and she'll keep on telling you …. (F9)

Male specific activities

There was overwhelming support amongst the fathers for all-male activities:

> I think I'd rather it be lads like—definitely—all men like. (F5)

> I prefer it [all men]—I do definitely—definitely. (F8)

Some believed that male-specific activities were vital to attract fathers in the first place:

> I mean it is crucial really that there's a dads club—if there wasn't a dads club solely I'm sure there's a lot of people wouldn't go to a mixed club.

> It's just the way men are. It doesn't bother me personally—but a lot of men won't go if it's mixed and stuff. (F3)

Several fathers gave detailed accounts of stressful experiences in mixed-gender sessions. One father recalled:

> I was like that when I first went to [one of the mixed groups]—I think there was only one other bloke there and meself and it was all women and they're all like looking at you—I was like running across the floor—you think 'oh God'—I was pleased when I went that the Fathers Worker was there—I was thinking 'I'll sit over here out the way' (laughing). (F8)

All eight mothers felt that an all-male environment was beneficial, some believing that it had helped their partners to take part in the first place. Examples of mothers' comments were:

> The fact that it is all men makes it easier for them to go—[my partner] won't go to anything mixed with me—it's a good idea for them to have their own stuff. (M5)

> The dads' club is great— [dads] do it because other dads are doing it. (M2)

High interest or 'hook' activities

Another important strategy was the use of high interest or 'hook' activities explicitly developed to appeal to men. The aim was to draw fathers into the programme and then to interest them in other sessions, once a positive relationship has been established. The development of such 'hook' activities required careful planning however, particularly when they did not appear to relate directly to the stated Sure Start aims and objectives. For example, it was important to emphasise that the Martial Arts class was not about 'fighting'; rather it used a range of sophisticated techniques to teach relaxation and anger management. A key member of staff stated that the programme has to offer services:

> ... which recognise the situation that men are in. If a man has a partner with Post Natal Depression, then the father is the key to that woman's well-being. If the woman is depressed, the father may also become depressed as well as the baby. There is a ripple effect. The courses they offer help men to think about their place in the family and their place in relation to other men.

The Martial Arts class was successful at a number of levels. Firstly, it has attracted large numbers of fathers into the programme. In both 2003 and 2004, it was the best attended activity, achieving a total of 191 attendances over the two years. The activity has appealed to a number of men. One father commented:

> If it was something like knitting or that kind of activity, I wouldn't have stuck it out but it's a masculine thing you know—I'm doing martial arts—that kind of thing. (F4)

It would appear that this strategy has been successful. The Martial Arts class accounted for 17% of male attendances in 2003 and 20% in 2004. Further, just under two-thirds of those whose first contact was through this class or through football went on to use other services.

Effective first contacts

Having first developed activities which were attractive to fathers and then persuaded them to take part, Sure Start Hinton's next step was to welcome and support them within the crucial first few sessions. If the father's experience was positive he was likely to return.

> The [Dads Worker] always get like new members involved as well—rather than you just being sat in the corner on your own just being quiet like you normally do when you don't

know people—when I first come like—I didn't know anyone—[the dads worker] was just constantly trying to get us involved. (F8)

The next stage in the retention process was to contact fathers, usually by phone, after they had attended their first group to ask for their views on the session and to encourage them to come again. Again fathers themselves commented on the worker's persistence in this regard:

She doesn't let go—she'll follow up and follow up and follow up .... (F6)

This 'on the spot' following up seemed essential in retaining father involvement. Again, it seems to be a proactive and assertive approach which achieved good results.

Strategies to keep men engaged

An important factor in keeping men involved was that the agenda for activities and events was user led. Several fathers commented that they had an opportunity to 'have their say' in terms of the activities and trips they could take part in.

Its not like [the worker] says 'look we're going to do this—we're going to do that'—we have an input in it—it's not just we're going to do this and nobody turns up—nobody's interested in it—you know. (F3)

[Staff] usually say that there's a range of things that we can do—usually geared to what fathers want rather than being based on someone else's idea—gives them more of an option. (F10)

One of the mothers we spoke to believed that involving men in decision-making was vital:

What works more than anything is that they can have a say. (M2)

Tensions and ways forward

As is to be expected, given the newness and scale of the task, Sure Start Hinton experienced a number of challenges in developing its work with fathers. Managers guiding the development of fathers' work were acutely aware that in order to expand and sustain fathers' involvement in future, responsibility for it must be shared across the whole team and between agencies. As one professional pointed out, the task requires 'a shift in organisational culture' since all staff may not have experience of the approaches and structures which are necessary to include men.

Lloyd *et al.*'s (2003) report on fathers work for the National Evaluation of Sure Start concluded:

To increase father involvement, it is essential that commitment to father involvement permeates the whole Sure Start programme ... A programme-wide commitment to fathers. (p. 52)

In order to include men fully, it was clear that there was a need for change at a number of levels which caused tensions in some areas. For example, there are differences in the ways that men and women interact in groups which some staff were more familiar with than others. The employment commitments of many men meant that more flexible patterns of staff working were required which had significant structural implications for staff working conditions. Such changes required on-going skilled negotiation on the part of the Programme's Manager.

Discussion

This study demonstrates how one Sure Start programme was able to engage large numbers of fathers with their early years services, in somewhat stark contrast to the majority of other local programmes, as noted above. Several of the approaches used by Sure Start Hinton to engage fathers are consistent with other strategies found to be effective in working with men, such as persistence in seeking fathers out and making services less female dominated (Ghate *et al.*, 2000), in addition to taking account of what motivates fathers (Lloyd, 2001). What singles Sure Start Hinton's work out as qualitatively different from that undertaken by others, is that many of those approaches found to be effective have been implemented within the context of relatively small scale projects (see Lloyd's (2001) study 'What Works with Fathers', for example). By contrast, Sure Start programmes, as forerunners of children's centres, were wide-ranging whole service delivery mechanisms for families across local neighbourhoods and as such, the success achieved by Sure Start Hinton has a number of important implications for the more widespread inclusion of men in early years services.

Firstly, the consistent use of a combination of both strategic and day-to-day strategies was fundamental to the programme's success in engaging men. At a strategic level, close day-to-day partnership working with an expert voluntary agency and the persistent use of a gender differentiated approach was perceived to be vital, as was on-going commitment to the work at programme management level. At a day-to-day level, the skills, abilities and persistence of the dedicated Fathers Worker, strongly supported by a dual management structure were fundamental to the work's continuing success. Having said this, whole staff training to support the development of a team-wide approach was found to be essential in working towards sustainable change in the delivery of all programme services to men. In addition, the implicit use of a social marketing strategy in which the views of fathers/male carers on what should be provided and how were gained on an on-going basis, with activities and events then 'sold' to fathers in a very proactive way, seemed particularly effective. Such an approach may be especially men-friendly since by taking consumer desires as its starting point, a social marketing strategy is likely to avoid difficulties with negative male perceptions of often used service terms, such as 'help', 'need' and 'support' (Summers *et al.*, 2004).

It is especially important that lessons from such effective work are learnt within a policy context which continues to introduce ever greater requirements for male involvement with family services. Practice Guidelines for Children's Centres (DfES, 2006) stated that:

All Sure Start Children's Centre services should be responsive to supporting fathers in their role as a parent and in their relationship with their partner or ex-partner, and more generally to promote the role of fathering. (p. 81)

Despite this much more explicit guidance on father engagement for children's centres than was initially produced for Sure Start local programmes, early indications on progress continue to be disappointing, with the National Audit Office concluding that centres were found to be *less effective at meeting the needs of fathers* (National Audit Office, 2006, p. 34).

Since the launch of children's centres, however, even greater obligations have been placed on public services to include men. Since April 2007, facilitating male access to services has become a matter of legal concern, with the introduction of the Gender Equality Duty which legally obliges all public bodies to:

Gather and use information on how the public authority's policies and practices affect gender equality in the workforce and in the delivery of services. (Equal Opportunities Commission, 2007, p. 3)

In practice, this means that men are now legally entitled to receive services in ways which best meet their needs and this represents a very important change in terms of accountability with regard to accessible service provision.

Sure Start Hinton's effective work in achieving father inclusion within their services demonstrates that high levels of male engagement can be achieved through the consistent and integrated use of both strategic and day-to-day approaches. Its efforts need to be replicated and extended at both local and national level, if men are to be more effectively supported in their fathering role. The task is a challenging one but the long-term benefits are likely to be great. As Carpenter (2002) noted:

In empowering fathers ... through inclusive practices, professionals can strengthen and empower the whole family network. (p. 201)

Finally, this is one father's vision of what might be gained through greater father access to men-friendly services:

We've found with the dads group—it's making them better people more interested, more interactive with their children—which makes them better children and as they grow up they'll pass it on and you've started the ball rolling—it's going to get better and better ....

Acknowledgements

The evaluation, of which this study was a component, was funded by the Sure Start programme as part of a government requirement for independent evaluation of its activities. We would like to thank the fathers and mothers who contributed their views, along with programme staff. The evaluation was conducted by the Durham University Centre for Applied Social Research and we wish to acknowledge the contribution of other members of the research team.

References

Carpenter, B. (2002) Inside the portrait of a family: the importance of fatherhood, *Early Child Development and Care*, 172(2), 195–202.

DfEE (Department for Education and Employment). (1999) *Sure start: a guide for second wave programmes* (London, HMSO).

DfES (Department for Education and Skills). (2003) *Every child matters* (London, TSO).

DfES (Department for Education and Skills). (2006) *A sure start children's centre for every community: phase 2 planning guidance, 2006–08* (London, HMSO).

Dubowitz, H., Black, M. M., Cox, C. E., *et al.* (2001) Father involvement and children's functioning at age 6 years: a multisite study, *Child Maltreatment*, 6, 300–309.

Equal Opportunities Commission. (2007) *Overview of the gender equality duty: guidance for public bodies working in England, Wales and Scotland.* Available online at: http://www.equality-human   rights.com/en/forbusinessesandorganisation/publicauthorities/gender_equality_duty/pages/genderequalitydutydocuments.aspx (accessed 17 December 2007).

Fagan, J. & Iglesias, A. (1999) Father involvement program effects on fathers, father figures, and their head start children: a quasi-experimental study, *Early Childhood Research Quarterly*, 14, 243–269.

Ghate, D., Shaw, C. & Hazel, N. (2000) *Fathers and family centres* (York, Joseph Rowntree Foundation).

Goldman, R. (2005) *Father involvement in their children's education* (London, NFPI).

Henricson, C., Katz, I., Mesie, J., Sandison, M. & Tunstill, J. (2001) *National mapping of family services in England and Wales* (London, National Family and Parenting Institute).

Lamb, M. (Ed.) (2004) *The role of the father in child development* (4th edn) (Chichester, Wiley).

Lewis, C. (2000) *A man's place in the home: fathers and families in the UK* (York, Joseph Rowntree Foundation).

Lloyd, N., O'Brien, M. & Lewis, C. (2003) *Fathers in sure start* (London, Sure Start Unit).

Lloyd, T. (2001) *What works with fathers* (London, Working with Men).

McDermott, R. J. (2000) Social marketing: a tool for health education, *American Journal of Health Behavior*, 24, 6–11.

National Audit Office. (2006) *Sure start children's centres.* Available online at: http://www.nao.org.uk/publications/nao_reports/06-07/0607104.pdf (accessed 17 December 2007).

O'Brien, M. (2004) *Fathers and family support: promoting involvement and evaluating impact* (London, National Family and Parenting Institute).

Robson, C. (2002) *Real world research* (Oxford, Blackwell).

Ryan, M. (2000) *Working with fathers* (Oxford, Radcliffe Medical Press).

Strauss, A. & Corbin, J. (1990) *Basics of qualitative research: grounded theory procedures and techniques* (London, Sage).

Summers, J. A., Boller, K. & Raikes, H. (2004) Preferences and perceptions about getting support expressed by low income fathers, *Fathering: A Journal of Theory, Research, & Practice about Men as Fathers*, 2, 61–83.

Tunstill, J., Allnock, D., Akhurst, S. & Garbers, C. (2005) Sure start local programmes: implications of case study data from the National Evaluation of Sure Start, *Children & Society*, 19, 158–171.

Why fathers are not attracted to family learning groups

Flora Macleod
University of Exeter, UK

Introduction

Provision of family learning opportunities does not in itself create a desire to become involved amongst both fathers and mothers, but especially fathers (Macleod, 2000). There is now a significant body of literature that makes clear that parental or family involvement in school means different things to mothers and fathers. This literature documents the gendered nature of the terms 'parent' and 'family' that positions mothers as the key parent in the success of their children's schooling (e.g. Lareau, 1989; Reay, 1998; Vincent & Warren, 1998; Crozier, 1999).

There are, of course, many factors that cause mothers to be positioned as the mainstream clientele for family learning programmes. Fathers, for example, not being resident in the family home as the number of female-headed households rise. But, even where fathers are present in the home, more mothers than fathers see it as their duty to know about their children's daily lives regardless of their work involvement. Findings such as these, which come from British Attitude Surveys conducted annually, are perhaps not surprising given that, only three decades ago, the norm was for mothers to be around the home and local area during the day looking after the children and maintaining the patterns and routines of everyday socialising within local communities. Although this is no longer the reality for many women, these norms and expectations for women, reinforced by both genders, are slow to change (e.g. Robertson et al., 2008).

Based on mounting evidence that father involvement has a positive impact on their children (e.g. Fagan and Iglesias, 1999; Lamb, 2004), there is much concern nowadays to acknowledge the crucial role of fathers in bringing up their children. This is apparent in recent UK government policies aimed at encouraging schools to make greater efforts to involve fathers in family learning and parental involvement activities. Despite this, all the available evidence points to the fact that fathers (defined to include biological fathers whether or not they are resident in the same home as their children, step-fathers and partners of women with children) are either reluctant attendees or, more usually, absent from family learning events (e.g. Ghate et al., 2000; Macleod, 2000).

The purpose of this paper is to explore this reluctance on the part of fathers from a social and cultural lifelong perspective by drawing on evidence from a national family literacy initiative. This perspective allows me to explore the complex issues that underpin the different responses of fathers and mothers to family learning provision. Crucially, by taking a cultural perspective the focus shifts away from conceiving low participation by fathers as a product of the barriers that individuals face onto long-term social processes as well as those that derive from the immediate context. To do otherwise is not to fully appreciate the nature of the problem.

Theoretical framework

I draw on Jerome Bruner's 1990 seminal work, *Acts of meaning*. Bruner's interest was in understanding *situated action*, that is, how we act in our everyday lives, the conditions for the action, and the constraints upon it. The main tenet of his theory, set out in *Acts of meaning*, is that our actions are not based on how things are, but on how we believe things should be. So as to give coherence to our lives and reconcile the irreconcilable, Bruner argues that our beliefs influence how we perceive things to be as opposed to how they actually are. His theory is an attempt to encapsulate how we live as we go about our everyday lives and the 'dispositions that characterize [us]: loyal wife, devoted father, faithful friend' (Bruner, 1990, p. 39). He suggests that when things in our lives are as they should be, that is in congruence with our beliefs, we have no need to explain or give reasons for our actions. However, when things are not as they should be, that is, there is an incongruence between how we perceive the state of the world around us to be and our beliefs such that we need to modify our plans and what we do, then we need to offer an explanation for our actions. This is because, according to Bruner, the world about us is not under our control, but what is under our control is how we respond. We can decide, for example, how what we do and plan to do based on our knowledge of what is appropriate and acceptable and what is inappropriate and unacceptable. Whilst the circumstances of our external worlds are not under our control, our actions are.

But, as the beliefs, rules, scripts and protocols under which we operate as we go about our daily activities are often implicit, we have to justify our actions retrospectively. For example, when asked why we acted in the way we did we give our reasons some time after the actions have occurred. According to Bruner, it is through this process of justifying what we do retrospectively, that we give coherent meaning to our actions. And, since justifying what we have done inevitably involves interpreting what we have done, our justifications are always normative and dependent on context. This means that the stories we create about what we have done are not only about justifying past actions but also about anticipating what we will do in the future. This, in turn, means that reasons for our actions are not only dependent on the rules and norms of our immediate context, but also on who we are, where we have come from. In this sense our actions are always dependent on our individual biography, our life history, including what we intend to do in the future, as well as the context in which the act took place. Our integrity thus needs to be taken account of in understanding the reasons for our actions. This is because we justify our actions in such a way as to ensure that it is not at odds with who we are.

Bruner sees the process of justifying our actions to ourselves and others as involving the construction of 'the longitudinal version of self' (Bruner, 1990, p. 120). This, in effect, means that the reasons we give for our actions can only be understood against the larger picture of our whole life which includes an anticipated future that inevitably will be constrained by the events we have experienced in the past. Although the reasons for our actions are given in the present, they are fused with past events which, in turn, are re-construed in the light of subsequent events. In other words, the reasons we give for or actions are inseparable from who we are, our identity.

One implication of taking this theoretical perspective to address empirical questions is to shift the focus away from the short-term experiences that might have shaped actions onto a life's past and future trajectory. A second implication is that the interest must be in exploring *reasons* for action rather than the *causes* of actions. Causes, as opposed to reasons, are more about the factors (internal and external to the person) that configure to bring about a certain outcome often from the 'objective reality' perspective. Whereas reasons puts the emphasis on folk psychology which is about people 'doing things on the basis of their beliefs and desires, striving for goals, overcoming, or not overcoming, obstacles, as they go along' (Bruner, 1990, pp. 42–43).

For Bruner, this is an important distinction. But for him the key difference is not so much between the external (objective) and internal (subjective) perspective but that in getting at *causes* we are about unravelling facts whereas in understanding *reasons*, fact and fiction become blurred. This is because the reasons (justifications) we give to ourselves and others for taking a particular course of action are contaminated by how we believe things should be or believe others think things should be. In this sense *reasons*, but not *causes*, are inevitably caught up in (implicit) social and cultural norms, scripts and protocols. Bruner maintains that any departure from the ordinary (what is normal and expected) to the exceptional requires a reason to be given. That is, an interpretation and justification is necessary to explain an incongruent action (an action that is out of step with what is appropriate or that would normally be expected). In this sense, when we justify our actions we not only recount them, we also give reasons that are morally, socially and psychologically acceptable to us and others for why we did what we did. This, in effect, means that we craft a personalised vision linked to a course of action we have taken or propose to take that has its source in the temporal and structural conditions of our lives as well as the immediate context of the action.

Using this theoretical perspective to help understand why fathers, but not their partners, were diverted away from family learning groups means exploring the reasons they give for their actions. This is because the reasons they give for attending, or, more usually, not attending would have made sense to them in terms of how they lived their lives in the past and intend to in the future, what they expect of themselves and what they felt was expected of them by others. This means that the reasons they gave for their actions were not just related to the immediate context of their lives, but also, in complex ways, to their biography. Although the action of attending or not attending took place at a particular point in time, this action, and the reasons given for it, were inseparable from who they were, where they had come from and what they planned to do in the future. Put simple, their self-identity—their integrity as a person over time—had to be taken account of when making sense of their actions.

Case study

The case study evidence used here comes from a UK-wide drive that targeted families with low basic skills and was supported by matched national and local funding. Whilst the initiative targeted families, it was, in practice, a place-based initiative. Like similar initiatives, families were targeted according to where they lived. They were identified through local schools which, according in certain indicators, were deemed to be serving socially and economically deprived areas. All families living in these areas were deemed to be considerably disadvantaged in terms of access to economic and social resources such as provision of adult learning to improve their prospect of employment and their general wellbeing. The initiative aimed to: provide family learning; encourage fathers to attend especially those who were neither employed or engaged in any other sort of adult learning; use the adult accreditation system to give the adult attendees formal recognition for their learning; encourage intergenerational learning through structured, relevant and enjoyable joint activities.

Whilst different approaches to delivery of family learning were encouraged, the main intervention model was made up of a 10-week programme of weekly sessions working with parents and their children in separate sessions followed by a joint session which brought them together to practise reading and writing. In the parent sessions there was a discernable adult education dimension to the programme which was normally led by an adult basic skills tutor. But, unlike many other adult education initiatives, these meetings were held in preschool or primary school settings during the school day so that they were in close proximity to their children to move straight into the joint (adult and child) family learning session. This meant that the recruitment of family members spanning two generations was in keeping with the intervention's intentions and fundamental to its success.

Despite one of the stated aims being to encourage fathers to attend, in the event, and in line with other such projects, mostly only women participated. Detailed case study data gathered from 18 randomly selected sites drawn from across the country showed that less than 2% of those who were recruited were men and all but one of these dropped out after one or two sessions. The parallel dropout rate amongst women was significantly lower. This was the case even though the men in the household appeared to be playing an important role in their children's daily lives. Often men could be seen, sometimes more so than women, being about the community during the day, pushing young children in buggies, dropping off and picking up older children at school, chatting and shopping locally with children in tow.

This was not surprising as, in many of the targeted communities, men were less likely than women to be at work as a result the decline of the manufacturing base in the UK. Although male unemployment tended to be high, there was plenty of low-paid, often part-time, work for women. Many fathers were therefore obliged to carry out tasks traditionally performed by mothers whilst their womenfolk worked. Yet, even though men had a regular presence at the school gate at the beginning and end of the school day, they showed little interest in participating in the family literacy programme. However, this high profile by uninvolved men meant that we were able to access their views with relative ease. Through numerous informal encounters and conversations with these uninvolved fathers, we gathered data on their reasons for not getting involved. It is these data that form the basis of this paper alongside interview data more formally collected through taped interviews from those who did attend, most of whom were mothers.

Across the 18 sites from which data were collected, a total of 163 women and 6 men attended at some point during the 10-week programme. Without exception the principal reason mothers gave for attending was to help their children with their school work and improve their own level of education and training. The handful of men who became involved, albeit briefly in five out of six cases, had various principal reasons other than this for being there. One father, a single parent, who attended with his new partner whom he had met at the school gate, wanted to gain custody of his child and was hoping that by attending he would get a good reference from his child's teacher.

In the event, from the 18 sites that provided data, he was the only father who stayed the course. Three of the other men were referred, along with their partners, by their local Social Service Departments. But, after the initial session, none showed up again even though their partners continued to attend. The remaining two men attended only briefly. One was newly cohabiting with a mother who attended and wanted to come along with her and the other was amongst the 'recently unemployed' and was looking for something to improve his skills, occupy his mind and fill up his days before being re-employed. Neither attended more than twice out of the 10 sessions and the recently unemployed male dropped out after the first. In both cases their partners continued to attend.

Most of the mothers said they preferred not to bring their own partner or husband with them and expected the other mothers to do likewise. Staff were also aware that mothers were not keen on having men present. Although their reasons were complex they included the desire not to bring 'couple issues' into the group. Unfortunately, we did not interview any of the five men who dropped out after they had left so we do not have their views on exactly why they left. Although we do have the views of two of them based on interviews conducted with them whilst they were attending. We evidenced that the attendance of men, however brief, had been a source of contention amongst some of the mothers. The two involved fathers we spoke to were both aware of this. They felt that if women were having problems with their partners the presence of men would make the group more tense. Early years' staff also mentioned in interview that the presence of men could make the group 'a scary place' for some women. By this they may also have been talking about themselves and their own feelings of being inhibited by the presence of men which is likely to have stemmed, at least in part, from the deeply feminine culture of their training (Colley et al., 2003; Hodkinson et al., 2007). The two briefly involved men and the uninvolved men we spoke to all said they felt ill at ease in a predominantly female environment. Some also said they felt tense in the presence of female staff as they sensed that they were nervous in their presence and unaccustomed to dealing with fathers.

The uninvolved fathers we spoke to, without exception, viewed the idea of a man attending family learning groups with suspicion. They believed that they would be regarded with suspicion if they showed interest in spending too much time hanging around a place where there were young children. They feared women and other men would suspect their motives. The suspicion of men who became involved was reflected in comments made by some of the mothers who attended and also members of the early years' staff who were responsible for running elements of the programme. Apart from the adult basic skills tutors who were accustomed to teaching mixed groups, generally it was felt that men who were attracted to this type of provision were in some way different to most men—usually this was in terms of their masculinity being open to question. According to the uninvolved men and some involved women, they were either hen-pecked by their womenfolk or (too much) in touch with their feminine side (not intended as a compliment). On the other hand, heterosexual males opting to attend were also not above suspicion as they might be preying on the women or, worse still, on *their* woman.

The strong focus on early years' activities (the family learning tasks on offer) were unattractive to men. As they saw themselves as practical and active they were not interested in participating in sedentary-type play activities with children or sitting around with women who were gossiping and drinking tea. Their preference was to participate in something more action-orientated activities such as going swimming or playing football. We were not able to investigate whether a change in the types of activities on offer would actually have made any difference. However, evidence from a different study suggests changes in the 'landscape for action' including the types of activities parent are expected to engage in can make school-based groups more attractive to men (de Rijke, 2005).

It seemed that any man daring to attend would risk being taken the wrong way by men, women and staff. For many mothers and fathers interviewed, any interaction between men and women was perceived as being potentially loaded with predatory intentions. Some fathers did not feel at ease talking to mothers at the school gate because it would make their own partner jealous and cause trouble. This potential for sexual tensions between men and women was frequently mentioned amongst the reasons given by mothers who preferred not to have their partners, or anyone else's, join the group. These mothers felt that if men were around they (the mothers) would need to present themselves differently by making more of an effort to dress nicely and put on their make-up. Also they believed men would inhibit the conversations that took place amongst mothers and between mothers and (female) staff. Part of what attracted these mothers was the opportunity the sessions provided for 'women's talk' and this would not be possible if men attended as well. A few women, staff and mothers, said they were uncomfortable in the presence of men and some mothers in female-only groups said they would probably leave the group if men joined it.

Those who stayed the course were rewarded for their efforts. We documented a range of benefits which included: an increased understanding of the ways in which they could support their children in literacy and language development and a better understanding of the relationship between home and school in children's education; an increased confidence and competence in providing more opportunities to interact with their children in the home around shared literacy activities; accreditation for adult learning and, in some cases, progression into further education, vocational training or employment. Although most programmes had a stronger focus on children's achievement, with less emphasis on parents' own learning, we documented examples of good practice in helping parents improve their own basic skills with related accreditation. Based on the information available to us, around 50% of the mothers and one father who attended the 18 sites studied, achieved accreditation of one sort or another by the time we had completed our fieldwork. This success, however, served to highlight the fact that the uninvolved had missed out on high quality local provision of adult and parent education. It is important, therefore, to gain a deeper understanding of the reasons why this sort of provision was unattractive to men. Although the focus of this analysis is on fathers, it is important to note in passing that this provision did not appear to be attractive to a significant number of mothers either.

Discussion

For the mothers who attended the family learning group meetings, the group became a shared public experience that gave them identity. The activities they engaged in were closely bound up in how they saw their role within the community as mothers and it fitted with how they wanted to be perceived by others. They had been brought up to take pride in fulfilling the role of mothering. But these same group meetings were regarded by many fathers, mothers and female staff, as 'no proper place for a man'. For the uninvolved men, it was alien territory and somewhat threatening. It was a feminised atmosphere that catered only for women. Attending would be an ordeal they preferred to avoid as it prevented them from being true to 'themselves' due to the 'femaleness' of the physical space. This 'hidden curriculum' manifested itself in the lack of male presence amongst staff and participants. The designers and providers of the curriculum were, without exception, women. Staff were without exception female and many admitted not having prior experience of working with men. Tasks/activities were heavily gendered. They were heavily rooted in 'mothering'. Fathers were expected to take on the role of both nurturing and teaching their young children. A process of putting men in touch with their feminine side. As the uninvolved men saw it, it was not just a matter of acquiring skills and competencies, as these were deeply embedded within the feminine culture but that attending was seen as a feminising process. Most men felt that this was not for them and most women felt that it was not for *their* men.

But most men, according to Ghate *et al.* (2000), feel, when given the option, they want time away from the family rather than time with them. Although a lot of women probably feel this too, they may be less inclined to say so publicly given the normative expectation of the mother's role. Even though these same men were quite content to be seen around the school at the opening and closing points in the day, chatting with one another and flanking the entrances, sitting around a table as part of a group mainly made up of women, drinking tea and gossiping, was not something they wanted either their womenfolk or other men to see them do. It was evident from this that none of the more superficial and easily removable barriers prevented them from attending, such as childcare, the time of day or being in work as few had any prospect of being in work. Childcare was provided and group meetings were conveniently tagged on to the beginning or end of the school day to make it possible for parents to attend without having to make a special trip.

The reasons for their non-attendance were much more deeply rooted than would be amenable to the 'quick-fix'. Uninvolved fathers and involved mothers had different preferences and priorities which were inseparable from who they were. Even though the environmental conditions around the uninvolved men had changed and the way they were spending their days had also changed from, for example, their fathers' generation, their justifications for their actions had not. This did not mean that they were not adapting or able to adapt to the changing conditions of their lives, they just preferred not to. Uninvolved men, spurred on by their partners and others around them, were crafting reasons for their non-attendance that defined themselves in relation to the group with which they identified.

In the one exceptional case of the male who stayed the course, the female staff and participants seemed quite relaxed in his presence. It is therefore of interest to consider why he was treated sympathetically and with less suspicion than was generally around/ towards (the prospect of) male attendees. Perhaps this was because he appeared to be comfortable in their presence and, as sole carer, did not have the choice of sending along his partner instead. But he too, like the men who were not there, had crafted a good story and one that fitted because it was linked to a course of action that he proposed to take which was socially acceptable. Female staff and participants were all made aware, as were we researchers, that he had an ulterior motive for being there (his desire to create a good impression in order to gain custody of his daughter) and we all seemed happy to support him in this venture. Also his (new) partner was present in the group so he neither fitted the stereotypical image of the male predator nor the feminised male. In this context he was quite happy to become 'one of the girls' for a short while and for his own very particular reasons. But this did not put him in a good position to help pave the way for other men to attend.

Seeing the lone male attendee as not being a pioneer means that those who see the attendance of one or two men as a step towards achieving father attendance in greater numbers are deluding themselves. Few men we spoke to aspired to be 'like' their female counterparts. Either they had to remain a 'real' man as defined by other men and women or become something else by blending into a female-dominated environment. But to do this would be in some way undermining or putting aside their masculine gender identity (Faulkner, 2000). The act of joining the groups would thus be problematic as it would indirectly imply that they had made a 'bad' choice or they were of the 'wrong' gender. To convey an image of being competent in the skills normally associated with motherhood would be hard to reconcile with their affinity with a male culture. Joining would mean they would have to balance their identities of being male and also doing women's work. The way the male who stayed the course did this was to put to one side for a temporary period only his concern to be 'one of the lads' and he had a socially acceptable justification for doing so. It would seem that the assumption that the isolated case of a father who attends will somehow and in some way point the way for a greater influx is a false conclusion. Rather, a fresh perspective is required that acknowledges the reasons (justifications) uninvolved and involved fathers give for their actions.

Trying to integrate fathers into existing provision is not a fruitful option as there is now convincing evidence that a 'mainstreaming, one-size-fits-all' approach just does not work. Instead greater gender sensitivity is essential. Whilst a handful of men may be prepared to distance themselves for short periods from masculinity and take on the norms of the dominant group, there is no evidence that the majority of men are willing to do so. If a male were to join family learning groups as they are currently conceived they would be seen not to fit the typical image of masculinity. Whilst the image for women in the reverse situation, the lone female in a male dominated environment, is often a strong and positive one, the reverse is the case for the lone male in a female-dominated environment. The problem, however, with dedicated provision appealing to men is that the script for family learning has already been written by women and the evidence is that both fathers and mothers are sticking to particular versions of their roles for normative reasons. The sense of what is right and appropriate and what is wrong and inappropriate is deeply engrained in men and women's biographies. For both the fathers and mothers we spoke to whilst conducting our fieldwork, this was a matter of normative judgement. This script is: 'women (mothers aspiring to become perfect) define the landscape for action, the tasks are designed by female early years' workers, and it is in this space that men are supposed to act out being a father'. The challenge for policymakers and practitioners is to re-write the script for father only groups rather than relying on only one template.

Conclusion

This paper was written in the context of UK central government concern to acknowledge the crucial role of fathers in bringing up their children. This concern, at least in deprived communities, has been extended to involving fathers in school-based family learning programmes. The dominant perspective here would appear to be that participation in these events by fathers is desirable and highly valued with little attempt to problematise the issue even though recruitment has been negligible. The conclusion that most research comes to is that, if men are to be engaged in family learning events in greater numbers, current strategies need to be modified (e.g. Ghate *et al.*, 2000). By shifting the focus from the individual onto the cultural, the conclusion of this analysis is more radical.

It has been argued that the reasons for the lack of interest amongst fathers lie in the apparent failure amongst researchers to appreciate fully the nature of the problem that they are addressing. Consequently, there has been much goodwill and tinkering at the edges. So long as the problem of low attendance by fathers is conceived of as an individual and institutional and not a cultural problem then the policy response will remain in the current vein. Researchers, like policymakers and practitioners, work within a social milieu where what they do is severely constricted by the political pressure to produce a 'quick-fix'. This reinforces the need to focus on that which is amenable to change such as timing of sessions, local provision and childcare issues and, consequently, can only give limited attention to addressing the deeply embedded feminine scripts of most family learning provision even though the available evidence suggests that the removal of barriers affecting individuals makes very little difference.

Looked at from a lifelong perspective, the picture that emerges is very different. Here father reluctance to attend is seen as the product of quite fundamental social processes that derive from their experiences in the wider social and cultural milieus of their lives. The analysis offers a direct challenge to relying solely on problem-focused policy research that is inclined to deal with the issue in isolation by assuming that individual and institutional factors can be separated from the social and cultural. In a sense, the call for greater father involvement is based on the claim that it is good because it is a desirable social value that all fathers should aspire to. This is in contrast to the more complex, but perhaps more appropriate; it is good because it is fulfilling for fathers, mothers, and children and, because of this, it can also make a difference to their social wellbeing.

Acknowledgement

The case study used here comes from research conducted with Neville Bennett, Louise Poulson and David Wray for the Basic Skills Agency.

References

Bruner, J. (1990) *Acts of meaning* (Cambridge, MA, Harvard University Press).

Colley, H., James, D., Tedder, M. & Diment, K. (2003) Learning as becoming in vocational education and training: class, gender and the role of vocational habitus, *Journal of Vocational Education and Training*, 55(4), 471–498.

Crozier, J. (1999) Is it a case of 'we know when we're not wanted'? The parents' perspective on parent-teacher roles and relationships, *Educational Research*, 41(3), 315–328.

de Rijke, J. (2005) *Citizen participation and democratic involvement: the case of parental involvement in schools*. Doctoral thesis, University of Exeter.

Fagan, J. & Iglesias, A. (1999) Father involvement program effects on fathers, father figures and their Head Start children: a quasi-experimental study, *Early Childhood Research Quarterly*, 14, 243–269.

Faulkner, W. (2000) Dualisms, hierarchies and gender in engineering, *Social Studies of Science*, 30(5), 759–792.

Ghate, D., Shaw, C. & Hazel, N. (2000) *Fathers and family centres* (York, Joseph Rowntree Foundation).

Hodkinson, P., Anderson, G., Colley, H. *et al.* (2007) Learning cultures in further education, *Educational Review*, 59(4), 399–413.

Lamb, M. (Ed.) (2004) *The role of the father in child development* (Chichester, Wiley).

Lareau, A. (1989) *Home advantage: social class and parental intervention in elementary education* (East Sussex, Falmer).

Macleod, F. (2000) Low attendance by fathers at family literacy events: some tentative explanations, *Early Child Development and Care*, 161(1), 107–119.

Reay, D. (1998) Class work: mothers' involvement in their children's primary schooling (London, UCL Press).

Robertson, D., Smythe, J. & McIntosh, I. (2008) *Neighbourhood identity: people, time and place* (York, Joseph Rowntree Foundation).

Vincent, C. & Warren, S. (1998) Becoming a 'better parent? Motherhood, education and transition, *British Journal of Sociology of Education*, 19, 177–193.

Predicting preschoolers' attachment security from fathers' involvement, internal working models, and use of social support

Lisa A. Newland[a], Diana D. Coyl[b] and Harry Freeman[a]

[a]University of South Dakota, South Dakota, USA; [b]California State University at Chico, California, USA

Over the past three decades, an increased interest in understanding the roles and experience of fathers has grown within several scholarly disciplines (e.g. developmental psychology, sociology, public policy). In addition, roles within families have changed in association with women's increased participation in higher education and the labor force, men's declining wages and the rise in the number of dual-earner households. Men's increased role in childrearing coupled with women's participation in the workforce have required adults to carefully consider how best to manage work and parental responsibilities (Cabrera *et al.*, 1999; Marsiglio *et al.*, 2000). To keep pace with these changes, it is important for researchers to reconsider men's contributions to child outcomes, such as attachment security, within contemporary family contexts that utilize co-parenting strategies and social support.

Definitions of father involvement

Cultural views and societal expectations of parenting roles often reflect changes occurring within families and the division of family responsibilities (Pleck, 1997). Contemporary two-parent (biological and blended) families as well as single-parent households place adult males within fathering contexts that typically require them to assume some, or all, parental responsibilities. In two-parent families, fathers' primary responsibilities have moved beyond the traditional roles of breadwinner and disciplinarian to include more direct physical care (Gerson, 1993; Coltrane, 1996). As fathering has evolved, researchers have attempted to examine the salient aspects of that experience, focusing on the amount of father involvement (quantity of time), sometimes with the benefit of longitudinal data (e.g. Hofferth *et al.*, 1997; Grossmann *et al.*, 2002), the level of involvement associated with children's ages (Yeung *et al.*, 2001; Wood & Repetti, 2004), barriers to involvement due to nonresidential status (Bruce & Fox, 1999), and maternal influences (Beitel & Parke, 1998; Allen & Hawkins, 1999; McBride *et al.*, 2005). Thus, a significant body of scholarly work has emerged on father involvement and fathers' influences on children's development (review: Tamis-LeMonda & Cabrera, 2002).

Scholars have also focused on the types and quality of father involvement that demonstrate the multidimensional nature of fathering (Lamb, 1997; Pleck, 1997). These dimensions include: cognitive and affective aspects (Palkovitz, 1997), social constructions of fathering roles (Marsiglio *et al.*, 2000), generative fathering and identity (Hawkins & Dollahite, 1997; Rane & McBride, 2000), and social capital perspectives (Amato, 1998). Lamb *et al.* (1987) proposed a model of three primary dimensions of father involvement: (1) *Engagement* during caretaking, play and leisure activities, (2) *Availability* of fathers to their children, and (3) *Responsibility* in which fathers directly manage, organize, and plan for their children's welfare and care. Attachment theory also provides another relevant approach to examining fathers' perceptions of their relationships with their children and the pathways through which father involvement influences children's development.

Father involvement and children's attachment

Bowlby proposed a 'monotropy principle' (1958, 1969/1982) in which an infant shows a strong genetic bias toward focusing their attachment behaviors toward a single, primary caregiver (typically the mother), and will consistently exhibit a strong preference for that particular individual when distressed. However, during the first year, most infants ordinarily become attached to one or more other individuals with whom they frequently interact—even if their interactions do typically not involve feeding or other needs-based caregiving. Thus attachment hierarchies develop, that include fathers and other family members (Bowlby, 1969/1982). Fathers have typically been associated with a secondary level of attachment relationships. However, recent studies have shown that fathers who participate in caregiving are more sensitive with their infants (Feldman, 2000; Roggman *et al.*, 2002), who in turn are found to be more securely attached to their fathers (Caldera, 2004). In addition, father responsiveness and sensitivity to their infants' behavior and their ability to engage their infants in dyadic interactions are associated with emotion regulation (Crockenberg & Leerkes, 2000).

Some scholars, including Bowlby (1969/1982), suggest that fathers and mothers may contribute in different but complementary ways to children's social, emotional and personality development (Caldera, 2004). Researchers have found that fathers' engage in more play than caregiving during infancy (Yogman, 1981) and the preschool period (Grossmann *et al.*, 2002); this finding is consistent in numerous cross-cultural studies (see review in Lamb, 2002). Though fathers are capable of providing sensitive and responsive infant care, they tend to be more involved as their toddlers' become more autonomous (Lamb, 1997, 2002).

Securely attached preschoolers continue to use their attachment figures as a secure base, however, parenting behaviors that accommodate preschoolers' growing autonomy and desire for greater exploration while providing encouragement and reassurance and also promoting secure attachment (Bretherton *et al.*, 2005). Paquette (2004, p. 193) described the emotional bond between fathers and children as an 'activation relationship' which develops primarily through physical play. This contrasts with the mother–child emotional bond in which mothers provide calming and comfort to children in times of distress. Paquette suggested that fathers' propensity for more active, physical play, and their tendency to encourage risk-taking while providing children with a sense of safety and security, encourages the development of obedience and competition skills in children. Volling *et al.* (2002) observed an association between fathers' highly arousing or stimulating play situations, and its effect on children's emotion regulation. Grossman *et al.*'s (2002) findings from their longitudinal study of German families suggest that fathers' role as an attachment figure during the preschool years may be 'to provide security through sensitive and challenging support as a companion when the child's exploratory system is aroused, thereby complementing the secure base-role of the mother as an attachment figure' (p. 311). In the context of Bowlby's view of attachment as a balance between attachment and exploratory behaviors (1979), Grossman *et al.* suggest that paternal play sensitivity and support are essential components that complement maternal caregiving sensitivity.

Contextual influences on parenting: adult attachment and social support

Studies of adult attachment and parenting behaviors indicate that adult internal working models (IWMs) and attachment styles are associated with parenting behaviors in theoretically predictable ways. Generally, these studies have shown that parents with secure internal models of relationships with their parents show more warmth and positive engagement with their children compared with insecure parents (e.g. Crowell & Feldman, 1988; Cohn *et al.*, 1992) and fathers who recall secure relationships with their parents are more sensitive and involved with their children (Cowan *et al.*, 1996). Grossman *et al.* (2002) also reported that fathers' caregiving quality was related to their own IWMs of attachment. More specifically, 'fathers who valued attachment relationships were found to be more sensitive, supportive, and appropriately challenging during play with their toddlers,' (p. 324). Other researchers have attributed stability of fathers' play sensitivity to relatively stable attachment relationships (Carlson & Sroufe, 1995; Thompson, 2000). Rholes *et al.* (1997) found that compared to securely attached individuals, insecurely attached individuals (avoidant or anxious) anticipated being easily aggravated by young children, advocated stricter disciplinary practices, were less confident in their perceived ability to relate to their future children, and expected to convey less warmth. Simpson (1999) reported that compared to secure- and insecure-anxious attachment styles, insecure-avoidant individuals anticipated less satisfaction from caring for young children. More distal social relationships (e.g. social support from extended family, friends, and religious organizations) may also facilitate positive father involvement and father–child attachment (Roggman *et al.*, 2002).

Co-parenting and shared childrearing beliefs

Positive features of the couple relationship (e.g. supportive communication and marital satisfaction) appear to enhance fathers' daily involvement with their children (Coley & Chase-Lansdale, 1999) and fathers' positive involvement has been associated with mothers' attitudes and beliefs about fathering (Allen & Hawkin, 1999; Matta & Knudson-Martin, 2006). Bretherton *et al.* (2005) suggest that bidirectional influences are likely 'in which good marital relations foster positive father involvement, and helpful father involvement, in turn, fosters good marital relations' (p. 248). Positive marital relationships have also been found to be predictive of children's secure attachment and fathers' psychosocial health and self-development (Byng-Hall, 2002; Palkovitz, 2002).

Maccoby *et al.* (1990) defined co-parenting as how mothers and fathers either support or undermine one another in their mutual parenting roles. Co-parenting, which is distinct from individual parenting style, can be measured on two dimensions: supportiveness and intrusiveness, and appears to be a proximal link accounting for the impact of the marital relationship on parenting (McHale & Alberts, 2003). Both co-parenting and the quality of the marital relationship contribute to the quality of the parent–child relationship (Floyd *et al.*, 1998; Caldera & Lindsey, 2006). Lindsey *et al.* (2005) found that parents with similar childrearing beliefs were likely to be more supportive of one another's parenting, and fathers tended to be more supportive in co-parenting than mothers. These findings suggest that the nature of dyadic and triadic relationships within the family is important for understanding preschoolers' attachment security.

Study purpose

This study contributes to the growing literature on father involvement by examining fathers' parenting behaviors as a mediator between their IWMs of attachment, use of social support, and preschoolers' attachment security. Specifically, this study explored:

(1) how fathering context, specifically fathers' attachment to others (parents and romantic partner) and use of social support (from friends, family and spiritual sources) were related to parenting behaviors,
(2) how parenting and co-parenting were related,
(3) how fathering context is related to children's attachment security, and
(4) whether fathers' parenting behaviors mediated associations between fathering context and children's attachment security.

Methods

Participants

Participants were 102 fathers of preschoolers between the ages of two and five (51.3% males, 48.7% females). Two data collection sites were used: a rural community in the Midwestern USA, and a suburban, culturally diverse community in the Southwestern USA. Of the combined samples, approximately 61% were Caucasian, 24% Hispanic, 12% African-American, and 3% reported 'other' ethnicities. Participants' reported annual family incomes in the following categories: <$20,000 annually (7%), $20,000–$40,000 (20%), $40,000–$65,000 (37%) and >$65,000 (36%). Participants' educational backgrounds also varied considerably, within the following categories: some or completed high school (21%), some college or a four-year degree (64%), and graduate or professional degree (15%). Approximately, 76% of families were two-parent households, 19% were mother- or father-only households, and 5% indicated that the child was living with relatives or adoptive parents. In all cases, the responding parent or guardian currently lived with the child at least part time.

Procedures

Research assistants recruited parents of preschool-age children within local communities who were willing to complete a questionnaire regarding family activities and relationships. Parents were asked to report on only one child even if other preschoolers resided in the home. Questionnaires were administered in the participants' homes by research assistants. Only father responses were used in this study.

Measures

Adult attachment scale. Participants completed an adapted version of the Adult Attachment Scale (AAS) (Simpson *et al.*, 1992) based on three attachment vignettes originated by Hazan and Shaver (1987). For this study, the Simpson *et al.* (1992) measure, containing 13 items, was expanded to 39 items asking respondents to rate their feelings toward: (1) their romantic partner or spouse, (2) their mother, and (3) their father (i.e. 13 items per relationship) using a five-point Likert response scale ranging from 1 = 'strongly disagree' to 5 = 'strongly agree.' Sample items from this adapted version included: 'I rarely worry about being abandoned by my romantic partner/spouse,' 'I'm not very comfortable having my mother depend on me,' or 'I find it difficult to trust my father.' Higher scores represented greater attachment security within each relationship. Separate scores for romantic partner/spouse, mother, and father were computed with reliability coefficients ranging from .88 to .96.

Use of social support. Parents rated 14 statements regarding their use of various types of social support from family members, friends, and faith-based activities or beliefs with a five-point response scale ranging from 1 = 'never' to 5 = 'always.' Items were extracted from the Family Crises Oriented Personal Evaluation Scales (FCOPES) (McCubbin & Patterson, 1981; McCubbin *et al.*, 1991). Separate scores were computed for use of social support in three areas: (1) Family support (five items, alpha = .75, e.g. 'When there is a problem, do you talk about it with relatives?'); (2) Friend support (five items, alpha = .73, e.g. 'When there is a problem, do you ask for encouragement or support from friends?'); and (3) Faith-based support (four items, alpha = .83, e.g. 'When there is a problem, do you ask for advice from a minister, a pastor, or spiritual advisor?').

Parenting behaviors. Parenting items assessed father involvement, parenting techniques, and co-parenting techniques. Collapsing these items into a total parenting scale was not warranted given the unique parenting features being measured; therefore, separate scales were constructed for: (1) father physical play, (2) consistency of parenting, (3) consistency of co-parenting, and (4) co-parenting behaviors. In addition, individual items were retained for data analysis purposes when they measured unique constructs such as discipline techniques or specific types of play.

Father physical play was measured using an adapted version of the engagement items in the national Early Head Start Research and Evaluation Project (see Cabrera *et al.* 2004). For the 10 items measuring physical, exploratory, or active play items, participants were asked: 'How many times per week do you get a chance to do each of the following activities with your preschool child?' Respondents rated the items on a six-point response scale ranging from 1 = 'rarely' to 6 = '5+ times per week.' A physical play scale was constructed by computing the average level of involvement across items which included: playing pretend games, playing outdoor games, playing blocks, playing with sand, water, dirt, or snow, helping the child with large motor activities such as bikes or slides, rough housing with the child, building or fixing something together (real or pretend), doing art activities together, dancing together, and teasing or joking with the child to get him/her to laugh. The alpha for this scale was .83. Individual items were also examined for hypothesized associations with attachment security, based on past research.

Parenting and co-parenting consistency were assessed with two scales, and items were rated on a five-point Likert scale. The first scale measured individual parenting consistency from day to day, using averaged responses to two items: 'In general, I tend to discipline my child using the same standards and guidelines from day-to-day'; and 'In general, I tend to discipline my child using the same techniques from day-to-day (time-out, spanking, removing privileges, etc.)' (alpha = .73). The second scale measured consistency of co-parenting using averaged responses to two items: 'In general, my partner and I tend to discipline our child using the same standards and guidelines'; and 'In general, my partner and I tend to discipline our child using the same techniques (time-out, spanking, removing privileges, etc.)' (alpha = .80).

Co-parenting techniques were measured with three items rated on a five-point Likert scale. Items included: 'When managing the household demands, my spouse (or romantic partner) and I usually parent and manage the house by... *sharing tasks or responsibilities/doing them together,... taking turns with household responsibilities and parenting,...and... giving each other a temporary break from responsibilities when neces-sary.'* An average response was computed across these three items, with a scale alpha of .74.

Parents' use of spanking was measured with one item: 'I spank my child at least once per week,' rated on a five-point Likert scale. This item was reverse coded for further analysis, such that higher scores represented 'rare use of spanking.'

Child's attachment security. The Attachment Q-Sort (AQS) (Waters & Deane, 1985) measures children's secure-based behaviours in their home environments by assessing a range of behaviours believed to reflect 'the smooth organization of, and appropriate balance between proximity seeking and exploration' (Posada *et al.*, 1995, p. 306). Typically, a Q-list, which is adapted from the Q-Sort, is sent to parents a week in advance of the Q-Sort administration to allow time for reflection on their children's behaviors. In this study, a short form Q-list consisting of 62 items was embedded within the survey instrument, and parents were asked to rate each item on a three-point response scale ranging from 1 = 'not like my child' to 3 = 'like my child.' The reliability coefficient for child attachment behaviors computed from the 62-item adapted Q-list was .80, with higher scores indicating greater child attachment security.

Data analysis plan

All data were collected and coded separately for the two data collection sites. The data sets were compared on predictor and outcome variables, and no statistically significant differences were found. Given the relatively modest individual sample sizes, both data sets were combined for all further analysis in order to increase the power and the representativeness of the sample. In addition, potential group differences for demographic variables (e.g. fathers' income and ethnicity) were examined for each predictor and outcome variable, and there were no statistically significant differences found. Therefore, demographic variables were not included as covariates in further analyses.

Parenting behaviors were examined as a mediator between fathering context and children's attachment security, following the procedures described by Barron and Kenny (1986). Pearson correlation and multiple regression analyses were conducted to test the following relationships: (1) prediction from the independent variables (fathers' IWMs and use of social support) to the mediators (parenting behaviors including father physical play, father consistency, co-parent consistency, rare spanking, and co-parenting behaviors, (2) prediction from the independent variables to the dependent variable (child attachment security), and (3) prediction from the independent variables to the dependent variable, controlling for the mediating variables (parenting behaviors). In a perfect mediating model 'the independent variable has no effect when the mediator is controlled' (Barron & Kenny, 1986, p. 1177).

Results

Descriptive statistics

Means, standard deviations, and inter-correlations are presented in Table 1. All scaled scores shown are averages across items within that scale. The average scale scores for fathers' IWM's were relatively high, with the highest mean being fathers' IWM of romantic partner; many fathers reported secure attachments within each relationship type (i.e. mother, father, partner). The average scale scores for social support were noticeably lower, suggesting that fathers do not always use the types of social support measured on this scale. These fathers relied most on family support. For physical play, fathers reported engaging in the types of active, physical, exploratory play measured on this scale about two to three times per week, and reported rough housing with their child three to four times per week. Parent and co-parent consistency scores tended to be quite high; fathers reported that they almost always use the same standards and techniques from day to day, and generally use the same standards and techniques as their parenting partner. Most fathers reported that they did not spank their preschooler once per week or more, although there was some variability for this item. Fathers generally agreed that they co-parent by sharing tasks, taking turns, or giving each other breaks in parenting. Average Q-list scores were quite high indicating that fathers' reported that their preschoolers demonstrated behaviors indicative of secure attachment.

Correlation coefficients

Table 1 shows the intercorrelations between fathering context, physical play, co-parenting consistency and behaviors, and child attachment security. There were moderate, positive intercorrelations among fathers' IWMs, with the IWMs of fathers'

Table 1.   Descriptive statistics and correlations

Parent variable	Mean	SD	1	2	3	4	5	6	7	8	9	10	11	12	13	14	15
									Fathering context (variables 1–6)								
1. IWM partner	4.52	.46	—	.39**	.35**	.15	.03	.18	.14	.21*	.12	.14	.17	.34**	.23*	.14	.37**
2. IWM mother	4.22	.61	.39**	—	.59**	.32**	.08	.04	.07	.09	.10	.01	.01	.11	-.10	.21*	.11
3. IWM father	3.96	.86	.35**	.59**	—	.18	.10	.08	-.06	-.03	-.03	.03	.01	.15	.10	.10	.15
4. Family support	2.84	.71	.15	.32**	.18	—	.39**	.16	.18	.16	.33**	.02	.10	-.08	-.04	.10	.14
5. Friend support	2.08	.66	.03	.08	.10	.39**	—	.44**	.37**	.20*	.27**	.22*	.01	-.22*	.13	-.01	-.05
6. Faith support	2.66	1.00	.18	.04	.08	.16	.44**	—	.17	.09	.09	.14	-.04	.12	.02	.08	.16
7. Active play	3.60	1.01	.14	.07	-.06	.18	.37**	.17	—	.58**	.68**	.61**	.17	.09	.26**	-.09	.15
8. Rough housing	4.76	1.37	.21*	.09	-.03	.16	.20*	.09	.58**	—	.46**	.22*	.23*	.29**	.13	.00	.30**
9. Pretend	3.60	1.66	.12	.10	-.03	.33**	.27**	.09	.68**	.46**	—	.24*	.05	.04	.12	.05	.26**
10. Build/fix	3.02	1.49	.14	.01	.03	.02	.22*	.14	.61**	.22*	.24*	—	.09	.06	.30**	-.08	.18
11. Parent consistency	4.55	.67	—	—	—	—	—	—	—	—	—	—	—	.33**	.28**	-.03	.28**
12. Co-parent consistency	4.36	.85	—	—	—	—	—	—	—	—	—	—	—	—	.27*	.19	.33**
13. Co-parent behaviors	3.72	1.58	—	—	—	—	—	—	—	—	—	—	—	—	—	.03	.21*
14. Rare spanking	3.68	1.05	—	—	—	—	—	—	—	—	—	—	—	—	—	—	.26*
15. Child security	2.39	.20	—	—	—	—	—	—	—	—	—	—	—	—	—	—	—

*p < .05, **p < .01

own parents being the most strongly correlated. There were also small to moderate intercorrelations among the social support scales, and among father physical play and co-parenting variables.

Research Q1 examined how fathering context, specifically fathers' IWMs of parents and romantic partner and use of social support, were related to parenting behaviors. Results indicate small to moderate positive associations of IWMs of romantic partner with father rough housing, co-parenting consistency and co-parenting behaviors. Associations of IWMs of mother and father with parenting variables tended to be small and non-significant, with the exception that fathers' IWMs of mother was positively related to fathers' rare use of spanking. Social support variables (family, friend, and spiritual) also had small to moderate associations with parenting variables. Friend support was most strongly related to all physical play variables, but was negatively related to co-parent consistency.

Research Q2 examined the extent to which fathers' parenting consistency and physical play would be related to co-parenting. As expected, there were small to moderate associations between co-parenting (consistency and behaviors) and fathers' consistency and physical play. Specifically, fathers' consistency was moderately related to both co-parenting consistency and behaviors. Rough housing was also related to co-parent consistency and father involvement in physical play and 'build or fix-it games' were related to co-parenting behaviors.

Research Q3 examined the relations between fathering context and children's attachment security. Findings shown in Table 1 indicate mostly small correlations between fathers' contextual variables and child attachment security. The strongest and only statistically significant correlation was between fathers' IWMs of romantic partner and child attachment security; small non-significant positive correlations of fathers' IWMs of parents with child attachment security were also observed. Friend support was weakly and negatively correlated with child attachment security, while the other social support scales were positively related to attachment security (although these were non-significant coefficients).

Research Q4 examined fathers' parenting and co-parenting behaviors as a mediator between fathering context and children's attachment security. Table 1 also shows small to moderate positive correlations between parenting behaviors and child attachment security, and all but two of these correlations were statistically significant. The strongest associations were between child attachment security and rough housing and co-parent consistency. In order to fully answer Research Q4, regression analysis was used to test the mediating effect of fathering on child attachment.

Regression analyses

Following procedures outlined by Barron and Kenny (1986), three sets of regressions were run to determine if parenting behaviors mediated associations between fathers' IWMs and their use of social support with child attachment security. To create the most parsimonious and predictive model while minimising problems with colinearity, the number of predictors in the model was limited. Based on theory, past research, and preliminary analyses, friend social support and fathers' IWM of romantic partner and mother were included in the model as independent variables, while rough housing play, parent and co-parent consistency, rare use of spanking, and co-parenting behaviors were included as mediators. Only the final model is presented in Figure 1, while intermediary steps are discussed next. Figure 1 shows the final path analysis model constructed from a series of regressions that were run to test the effects of fathering context on fathering behaviors, the effect of fathering context on child attachment security, and the effects of fathering context when controlling for fathering and co-parenting behaviors. *F*-values and significance levels are shown above each dependent variable for each regression, and Beta weights and significance levels are shown for each path. As shown in the path model, a series of regressions tested the prediction from fathering context to fathering and co-parenting behaviors, and all of those models were statistically significant (see Figure 1). Fathering context (IWM mother, IWM romantic partner, friend support) did predict child attachment security (F = 5.58, p = .001), but the only significant predictor in the model was IWM romantic partner (β = .40, t = 3.89, p = .000, not shown in final model). Fathering and co-parenting behaviors also uniquely predicted child attachment security (F = 5.46, p = .001), with the strongest fathering predictors being rare spanking and rough housing play (not shown). Lastly, the mediators were included in a stepwise model predicting child attachment security from: Step 1 fathering context and Step 2 context while controlling for parenting. In the final model, IWM of romantic partner remained a unique predictor of child attachment security, even while controlling for fathers' play, discipline, and co-parenting, suggesting that parenting does not completely mediate associations between context and child attachment security. However, rough housing play remained a statistically significant unique predictor of attachment security while controlling for fathering context, and the path coefficient was higher than that for fathers' rare spanking, consistency, and co-parenting consistency and behaviors, suggesting that father play adds unique predictive power when predicting preschooler attachment security.

Discussion

This study complements previous research on fathers' influence on young children's attachment security. Specifically, we examined relations between contextual parenting variables (fathers' IWMs and social support), specific parenting behaviors, and co-parenting. In addition, we tested proximal parenting behaviors as a mediator between fathers' social support, IWMs and their preschooler's attachment security. Our findings suggest that fathers' IWMs and use of some types of social support were related to parenting and co-parenting behaviors, and these in turn were predictive of child attachment security. Father play, consistency and discipline were related to co-parenting consistency and behaviors, indicating inter-relatedness between fathering and co-parenting. Fathers' IWM of partner was predictive of child attachment security, and remained so, even when controlling for parenting behaviors (although the

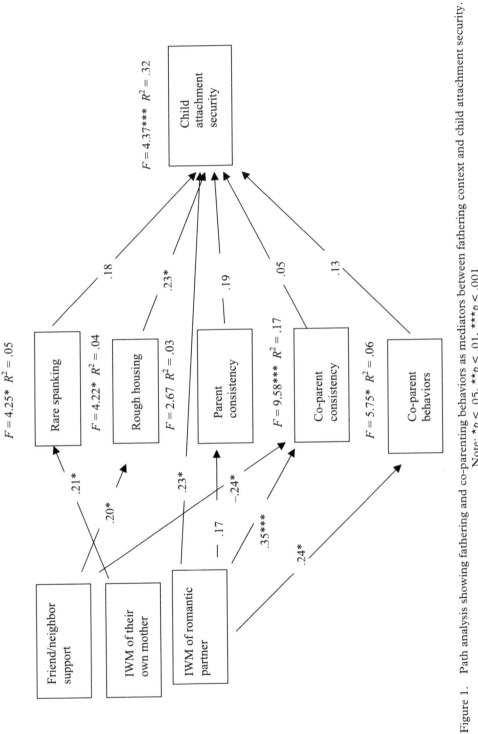

Figure 1. Path analysis showing fathering and co-parenting behaviors as mediators between fathering context and child attachment security.
Note: $*p < .05$, $**p < .01$, $***p < .001$

predictive power decreased when parenting was included in the model, suggesting mediation through parenting). Several parenting and co-parenting factors were related to child attachment security, but when they were included together with fathering context, only one fathering variable, rough housing, remained as a significant predictor of child attachment security. Thus, rough housing play was more predictive of child attachment security than were father sensitivity (non-physical punishment) and consistency. This is consistent with Paquette's (2004) notion that the bond between father and child develops through physical play.

These findings are also consistent with Byng-Hall's (2002) premise of a secure family base, in which the child(ren) and parents all have access to emotional support which leads to felt security for each family member. Fathers who are secure in close relationships, particularly with their partner, are more likely to use consistent and responsive parenting practices including active play involvement with their preschoolers (Belsky, 1999; Coley & Chase-Lansdale, 1999; Simpson, 1999; Frosch et al., 2000). In this study, fathers with more secure IWMs of their mothers, and who utilised family support, were more likely to be involved with their preschooler and were less likely to use physical punishment as a discipline strategy, suggesting that their felt security is important for maintaining positive father–child relationships. Fathers' use of friend support was also found to be related to a number of father involvement activities, but was negatively related to co-parenting consistency. This warrants further investigation as to how and why fathers' friends may support father–child involvement, but not co-parent consistency. It may be that father reliance on friend support hinders closeness and consistency with their parenting partner. Associations between fathers' IWM of partners, co-parenting, and child attachment security are in line with previous research which suggests that marital relationship quality predicts co-parenting consistency and child attachment security (Bretherton et al., 2005).

Father physical play, parenting consistency, and co-parenting seem to operate in conjunction with one another as proximal processes which benefit the father–child attachment relationship. Even so, rough housing emerged as a unique predictor of child attachment security, above and beyond other parenting and co-parenting behaviors. These results suggest that fathers' physical play involvement provides a unique contribution to young children's attachment security (Bowlby, 1969/1982; Grossmann et al., 2002; Paquette, 2004; Bretherton et al., 2005).

The strengths of this study include the use of a diverse (i.e. income, education levels, and ethnicity) non-clinical sample of fathers from two-parent and single-parent households and from two distinct regions in the USA. We measured several family process and contextual variables which have been theoretically linked to children's attachment security, and in some cases previously tested empirically. Despite these strengths, the study has several limitations. The sample, though diverse on a number of indicators, was relatively small when compared to the number of US families with preschoolers. Further studies with larger father samples from other countries as well as from the USA would help determine whether the results of this study were replicable.

Limitations associated with data collection include the measurement of all variables via a questionnaire. The current measure of adult attachment may not fully capture the complexity of adult IWMs. Interviews with fathers could facilitate more candid and richer information regarding their history of attachment relationships, parenting beliefs, behaviors and co-parenting. Given the potential importance of specific types of father activities in supporting children's attachment security, the development and testing of reliable and valid measures of physically active or arousing types of play is warranted. Direct observation of fathers' physical play with preschoolers might also yield more in-depth knowledge of how father–child activities, parenting techniques and behaviours affect young children's attachment security. Further studies could expand on this work by triangulating measures and including interviews with mothers and fathers as well as observational data. Gathering data on multiple proximal and context variables would be useful to better understand functional family systems that support children's attachment within a secure family base.

Findings from this study may be useful for practitioners who work in early childhood education and community agencies that serve parents and children, particularly agencies focused on fostering father involvement. Parent education, modeling, or mentoring from father educators or other family professionals should include: (1) the acknowledgment of the important contribution fathers make to their children's attachment security, (2) the encouragement of shared father–child activities and non-punitive forms of guidance, (3) Parenting consistency, and (4) the establishment or reinforcement of co-parenting behaviors. Our study findings suggest that the support of father involvement in physical play activities, co-parenting consistency and behaviors, and non-punitive forms of guidance foster young children's attachment security. Yet, just as importantly, our findings call into question parenting interventions that focus solely on parenting behaviors without taking into account parent gender and the context in which parenting occurs (e.g. the quality of the marital relationship, and support from sources such as family and friends).

Practitioners who address fathers' well being, particularly the quality of the marital or partner relationship, will likely capture more of the family ecology responsible for children's attachment security. Parenting context within individual families could include the availability or use of social support as another indirect but potentially important influence on fathers' involvement, particularly in father-only families. Mothers might also benefit from understanding the importance of supporting fathers' involvement as a benefit not only to father–child relationships, but also to the marital relationship. Facilitating supportive, responsive interactions among fathers, mothers, and children will likely sustain or help create secure relationships among all family members.

References

Allen, S. M. & Hawkins, A. J. (1999) Maternal gatekeeping: mothers' beliefs and behaviors that inhibit greater father involvement in family work, *Journal of Marriage and the Family*, 61, 199–212.

Amato, P. (1998) More than money? Men's contributions to their children's lives, in: A. Booth & A. C. Crouter (Eds) *Men in families: when do they get involved? What difference does it make?* (Mahwah, NJ, Lawrence Erlbaum), 241–278.

Barron, R. M. & Kenny, D. A. (1986) The moderator-mediator variable distinction in social psychological research: conceptual, strategic, and statistical considerations, *Journal of Personality and Social Psychology*, 51(6), 1173–1182.

Beitel, A. H. & Parke, R. D. (1998) Paternal involvement in infancy: the role of maternal and paternal attitudes, *Journal of Family Psychology*, 12, 268–288.

Belsky, J. (1999) Interactional and contextual determinants of attachment security, in: J. Cassidy & P. R. Shaver (Eds) *Handbook of attachment: theory, research, and clinical applications* (New York, Guilford), 249–264.

Bowlby, J. (1958) The child's tie to his mother, *International Journal of Psycho-Analysis*, 39, 350–373.

Bowlby, J. (1969/1982) *Attachment and loss. Vol. 1: attachment* (2nd edn) (New York, Basic Books).

Bowlby, J. (1979) *The making and breaking of affectional bonds* (London, Tavistock).

Bretherton, I., Lambert, J. D. & Golby, B. (2005) Involved fathers of preschool children as seen by themselves and their wives: accounts of attachment, socialization, and companionship, *Attachment and Human Development*, 7(3), 229–251.

Bruce, C. & Fox, G. L. (1999) Accounting for patterns of father involvement: age of child, father-child coresidence, and father role salience, *Sociological Inquiry*, 69, 458–476.

Byng-Hall, J. (2002) Relieving parentified children's burdens in families with insecure attachment patterns, *Family Processes*, 41(3), 375–388.

Cabrera, N. J., Shannon, J. D., Vogel, C. *et al.* (2004) Low-income fathers' involvement in their toddlers' lives: biological fathers from the Early Head Start Research and Evaluation Study, *Fathering*, 2, 5–30.

Cabrera, N. J., Tamis-LeMonda, C., Lamb, M. E. & Boller, K. (1999) Measuring father involvement in the Early Head Start evaluation: a multidimensional conceptualization, paper presented at the *National Conferences on Health Statistics*, Washington, DC, September.

Caldera, Y. M. (2004) Paternal involvement and infant-father attachment: a Q-set study, *Fathering*, 2, 191–210.

Caldera, Y. M. & Lindsey, E. W. (2006) Coparenting, mother-infant interaction, and infant-parent attachment relationships in two-parent families, *Journal of Family Psychology*, 20(2), 275–283.

Carlson, E. & Sroufe, L. A. (1995) The contribution of attachment theory to developmental psychology, in: D. Cicchetti & D. Cohen (Eds) *Developmental processes and psychopathology, Vol. 1: theoretical perspectives and methodological approaches* (New York, Cambridge University Press), 581–617.

Cohn, D. A., Cowan, P. A., Cowan, C. P. & Pearson, J. (1992) Mothers' and fathers' working models of childhood attachment relationships, parenting styles, and child behavior, *Development and Psychopathology*, 4, 417–431.

Coley, R. L. & Chase-Lansdale, P. L. (1999) Stability and change in paternal involvement among urban AA fathers, *Journal of Family Psychology*, 13, 416–435.

Coltrane, S. (1996) *Family man: fatherhood, housework, and gender equity* (New York, Oxford University Press).

Cowan, P. A., Cohn, D. A., Cowan, C. P. & Pearson, J. L. (1996) Parents' attachment histories and children's externalizing and internalizing behaviors: exploring family systems models of linkage, *Journal of Consulting and Clinical Psychology*, 64, 54–63.

Crockenberg, S. & Leerkes, E. (2000) Infant social and emotional development in family context, in: C. H. Zeanah (Ed.) *Handbook of infant mental health* (New York, Guilford), 60–90.

Crowell, J. A. & Feldman, S. (1988) Mothers' internal models of relationships and children's behavioral and developmental status: a study of mother-child interaction, *Child Development*, 59, 1273–1285.

Feldman, R. (2000) Parents' convergence on sharing and marital satisfaction, father involvement, and parent-child relationship at the transition to parenthood, *Infant Mental Health Journal*, 21, 176–191.

Floyd, F. J., Gilliom, L. A. & Costigan, C. L. (1998) Marriage and the parenting alliance: longitudinal prediction of change in parenting perceptions and behaviors, *Child Development*, 69, 1461–1479.

Frosch, C. A., Mangelsdorf, S. C. & McHale, J. L. (2000) Marital behavior and the security of preschooler-parent attachment relationships, *Journal of Family Psychology*, 14(1), 144–161.

Gerson, K. (1993) *No man's land: men's changing commitments to family and work* (New York, Basic Books).

Grossmann, K., Grossmann, K. E., Fremmer-Bombik, E. *et al.* (2002) The uniqueness of the child-father attachment relationship: father's sensitive and challenging play as a pivotal variable in a 16-year longitudinal study, *Social Development*, 11, 307–331.

Hawkins, A. J. & Dollahite, D. C. (1997) *Generative fathering: beyond de?cit perspectives* (Thousand Oaks, CA, Sage).

Hazan, C. & Shaver, P. R. (1987) Romantic love conceptualized as an attachment process, *Journal of Personality and Social Psychology*, 52, 511–524.

Hofferth, S. L., Yeung, W. J. & Stafford, F. (1997) *Panel study of income dynamics*. Available online at: PSID website, http://www.isr.umich.edu/src/psid/index.html (accessed 15 February 2008).

Lamb, M. E. (1997) *The role of the father in child development* (3rd edn) (New York, John Wiley).

Lamb, M. E. (2002) Infant-father attachments and their impact on child development, in: C. Tamis-LeMonda & N. Cabrera (Eds) *Handbook of father-involvement* (Hillsdale, NJ, Lawrence Erlbaum), 93–117.

Lamb, M. E., Pleck, J. H., Charnov, E. L. & Levine, J. A. (1987) A biosocial perspective on paternal involvement, in: J. Lancaster, J. Altmann, A. Rossi & L. Sherrod (Eds) *Parenting across the lifespan: biosocial dimensions* (New York, Aldine de Gruyter), 111–142.

Lindsey, E. W., Caldera, Y. & Colwell, M. (2005) Correlates of coparenting during infancy, *Family Relations*, 54, 346–359.

Maccoby, E., Depner, C. & Mnookin, R. (1990) Co-parenting in the second year after divorce, *Journal of Marriage and the Family*, 52, 141–155.

Marsiglio, W., Amato, P., Day, R. D. & Lamb, M. E. (2000) Scholarship on fatherhood in the 1990s and beyond, *Journal of Marriage and Family*, 62, 1173–1191.

Matta, D. S. & Knudson-Martin, C. (2006) Father Responsivity: couple processes and the construction of fatherhood, *Family Processes*, 45, 19–37.

McBride, B., Brown, G., Bost, K., Shin, N., Vaughn, B. & Korth, B. (2005) Paternal identity, maternal gatekeeping, and father involvement, *Family Relations*, 54, 360–37.

McCubbin, H. I., Olson, D. H. & Larson, A. S. (1991) FCOPES: Family Crisis oriented Personal Evaluation Scales, in: H. I. McCubbin & A. I. Thompson (Eds) *Family assessment inventories for research and practice* (Madison, WI, University of Wisconsin-Madison), 193–207.

McCubbin, H. I. & Patterson, J. M. (1981) *Systematic assessment of family stress, resources, and coping: tools for research, education, and clinical intervention* (St Paul, MN, Department of Family Social Science).

McHale, J. & Alberts, A. (2003) Thinking three: coparenting and family-level considerations for infant mental health professionals, *Signal*, 11, 1–11.

Palkovitz, R. (1997) Reconstructing involvement: expanding conceptualizations of men's caring in contemporary families, in: A. J. Hawkins & D. C. Dollahite (Eds) *Generative fathering: beyond de?cit perspectives* (Thousand Oaks, CA, Sage), 200–216.

Palkovitz, R. (2002) *Involved fathering and men's adult development: provisional balances* (Mahwah, NJ, US, Lawrence Erlbaum Associates Publishers).

Paquette, D. (2004) Theorizing the father-child relationship: mechanisms and developmental outcomes, *Human Development*, 47, 193–219.

Pleck, J. (1997) Paternal involvement: levels, sources, and consequences, in: M. E. Lamb (Ed.) *The role of the father in child development* (3rd edn) (New York, John Wiley), 66–103.

Posada, G., Gao, Y., Wu, F., Posada, R., Tascon, J., Schoelmerich, A., Sagi, A., Kondo-Ikemura, K., Haaland, W. & Synnevaag, B. (1995) The secure base phenomenon across cultures: children's behavior, mother's preferences, and experts' concepts, in: E. Waters, B. E. Vaugh, G. Posada & K. Kondo-Ikemura (Eds) Caregiving, cultural, and cognitive perspectives on secure-base behavior and working models, *Monographs of the Society for Research in Child Development*, 60(2–3, Serial No. 244), 27–48.

Rane, T. R. & McBride, B. A. (2000) Identity theory as a guide to understanding fathers' involvement with their children, *Journal of Family Issues*, 21, 347–366.

Rholes, W. S., Simpson, J. A., Blakely, B. S., Lanigan, L. & Allen, E. A. (1997) Adult attachment styles, the desire to have children, and working models of parenthood, *Journal of Personality*, 65(2), 357–385.

Roggman, L. A., Boyce, L. K., Cook, G. A. & Cook, J. (2002) Getting dads involved: predictors of father involvement in Early Head Start and with their children, *Infant Mental Health Journal*, 23, 62–78.

Simpson, J. A. (1999) Attachment theory in modern evolutionary perspective, in: J. Cassidy & P. R. Shaver (Eds) *Handbook of attachment: theory, research, and clinical applications* (New York, Guilford), 115–140.

Simpson, J. A., Rholes, W. S. & Nelligan, J. S. (1992) Support-seeking and support-giving within couple members in an anxiety-provoking situation: the role of attachment styles, *Journal of Personality and Social Psychology*, 62, 434–446.

Tamis-LeMonda, C. S. & Cabrera, N. (Eds) (2002) *Handbook of father involvement: mutlidisciplinary perspectives* (Mahwah, NJ, Lawrence Erlbaum).

Thompson, R. A. (2000) The legacy of early attachments, *Child Development*, 71, 145–152.

Volling, B. L., McElwain, N. L., Notaro, P. C. & Herrera, C. (2002) Parents' emotional availability and infant emotional competence: predictors of parent-infant attachment and emerging self-regulation. *Journal of Family Psychology*, 16(4), 447–465.

Waters, E. & Deane, K. (1985) Defining and assessing individual differences in attachment relationships: Q-methodology and the organization of behavior in infancy and early childhood, in: I. Bretherton & E. Waters (Eds) Growing points of attachment theory and research, *Monographs of the Society of Research in Child Development*, 50(1–2, Serial no. 209), 41–65.

Wood, J. J. & Repetti, R. L. (2004) What gets dad involved? A longitudinal study of change in parental child caregiving involvement, *Journal of Family Psychology*, 18, 237–249.

Yeung, W. J., Sandberg, J. F., Davis-Kean, P. E. & Hofferth, S. L. (2001) Children's time with fathers in intact families, *Journal of Marriage and Family*, 63, 136–154.

Yogman, M. W. (1981) Games mothers and fathers play with their infants, *Infant Mental Health Journal*, 2, 241–248.

Father beliefs as a mediator between contextual barriers and father involvement

Harry Freeman[a], Lisa A. Newland[a] and Diana D. Coyl[b]

[a]University of South Dakota, South Dakota, USA; [b]California State University at Chico, California, USA

Nearly a century of research has established that children do better in school when their parents take an active role in their child's day-to-day learning (see Hess *et al.*, 1984; Coleman, 1991; Epstein, 1991; Kellaghan *et al.*, 1993; Muller & Kerbow, 1993; Hoover-Dempsey *et al.*, 2005 for reviews of this research). Although the first 50 years of research on parental involvement focused almost exclusively on mothers; a series of studies beginning in the 1970s demonstrate that fathers are a potent social force in the educational lives of children from infancy through adolescence (see

Amato & Rivera, 1999; Cabrera *et al.*, 2000; Lamb, 2004 for reviews). The question today for scholars, researchers, and policymakers is less about whether or not fathers are important to children's academic success, and more about understanding factors that contribute to father involvement, particularly among families in which men's participation with children is limited or constrained (Bruce & Fox, 1999; McBride *et al.*, 2005). The importance of supporting fathering involvement may be greatest among low-income populations, where limited education, inflexible work schedules, and restricted access to extra-familial social support are frequent barriers to parental involvement (Roggman *et al.*, 2002; Cabrera *et al.*, 2004). Identifying predictors of father involvement among low-income or at-risk families is critical to the success of early intervention programs, and is the subject of the current investigation (Grolnick *et al.*, 1997; Boller *et al.*, 2006; Brannen & Nilsen, 2006).

As a group, families living below the poverty level typically measure lower on parental involvement compared to higher-income families; however, within-group variation is considerably larger than between-group variation based on income categories (see Hoover-Dempsey *et al.*, 2005). In other words, income level does not explain *why* parents become involved. Rather, income and social status may represent barriers to involvement for low-income families. Barriers, in turn, may shape parents' beliefs about their capacity to become involved and to positively affect their child's development (Hoover-Dempsey & Sandler, 1997). We test this view in the current study by examining whether parenting beliefs mediate the connection between contextual barriers (e.g. work schedules and stress) and involvement among fathers enrolled in Head Start (HS) and Early Head Start (EHS) programs. By encouraging parent participation, HS and EHS programs hope to build positive parental beliefs that reinforce what fathers already know or can do through empowerment-based interventions. This intervention approach is consistent with the idea that fathers' beliefs are a more proximal and powerful influence on their actual involvement practices than family context and perceived barriers within that context. We hypothesise that pro-active father beliefs will predict involvement and, at the same time, diminish the explanatory power of contextual barriers.

The breadth of research covering parent involvement, as well as the more recent studies on father involvement, both contribute to a greater understanding of how family context explains father involvement. Contextual variables found to correlate with father involvement include: educational attainment, father age, family structure, parents' work schedules, mothers' age, autonomy, and occupation (Grossman *et al.*, 1988; Kissman, 2001; Matta & Knudson-Martin, 2006), maternal attitudes and beliefs about fathering including maternal gate-keeping (e.g. Beitel & Parke, 1998; Allen & Hawkins, 1999), marital conflict, biological relationship to child, extra-familial social support (Roggman *et al.*, 2002; Cabrera *et al.*, 2004), post-divorce parental conflict, visitation issues (King & Heard, 1999), and boundary ambiguity (Madden-Derdich *et al.*, 1999). These variables are typically examined as barriers to fathers' involvement. For instance, family structure is usually studied as father absence, fatherlessness, non-resident fathers, or more recently fragile family contexts (see King, 1994; Amato & Gilbreth, 1999; Garcia Coll *et al.*, 2002; Weiss *et al.*,

2003). A recent and extensive evaluation study of father involvement in EHS programs reported a higher rate of father–child interaction among non-resident fathers than indicated by previous reports. The authors suggested that many non-resident fathers are successful in staying involved in their child's life, especially when conflict with the child's mother is minimal. Understanding the complex or synergistic effect of multiple barriers may be approximated using a multiple risk factor model (Olson *et al.*, 2002; Brotman *et al.*, 2003). Rather than partialing out the variance of each barrier, adding them incorporates the cumulative effect of multiple stressors operating at the same time, an approach employed in the current study.

Household income is negatively associated with barriers, such that as income drops the number and intensity of barriers is likely to rise (Collignon *et al.*, 2001; Horvat *et al.*, 2003). Given the associations between SES and barriers it is clear why parent involvement, and more recently father involvement, is an integral component to most early intervention programs. HS and EHS strongly encourage parent participation in virtually all aspects of the program, from policy decisions to daily classroom activities; as program funding is tied to parents' involvement, multiple incentives are available for parents to become involved. The U.S. Department of Health and Human Services recently launched initiatives specifically targeting low-income fathers such as 'The National Head Start Institute on Father Involvement' which was created to improve opportunities for fathers to participate in the lives of HS children. In the early 1990s HS programs implemented a number of demonstration projects in the USA to increase the involvement of residential and non-residential fathers with their preschoolers (Fagan & Iglesias, 1999). Initial studies indicated that changing fathers' and mothers' attitudes about father involvement coupled with an emphasis on teaching specific parenting skills were more likely to enhance father–child relationship qualities (Fagan & Stevenson, 2002). Creating opportunities for parents to become involved in their child's education is believed to foster parents' beliefs regarding their role and influence in their child's development (Hoover-Dempsey & Sandler, 1997). In their model, Hoover-Dempsey and Sandler identify two categories of beliefs, parental role construction and self-efficacy, as most proximal to involvement practices.

Parents' role construction identifies parents' beliefs about activities within the home and school that parents deem as 'important, necessary, and permissible' to their child's learning (Hoover-Dempsey & Sandler, 1997, p. 17). In assessing this construct, parents are asked to rate the extent to which they believe the responsibility for their child's learning is charged to parent activities, teacher activities, and activities which involve both parents and teachers. The importance of role construction to parent participation is supported by a number of recent studies (Hoover-Dempsey *et al.*, 2005; Green *et al.*, 2007), and the effect appears robust with respect to ethnic, geographic, and SES diversity (Green *et al.*, 2007). Equally important, role construction is amenable to interventions across diverse family contexts (Fagan & Stevenson, 1995, 2002). In the current study, questions were included to measure fathers' beliefs about their role in their child's education and caretaking and their perceived responsibility to the HS/EHS program specifically (responsibility to program).

Parents' *sense of efficacy for helping children succeed in school* comprises the second category of beliefs in Hoover-Dempsey and Sandler's model. This construct indexes the extent to which parents believe their involvement 'can exert a positive influence on children's educational outcomes' (Hoover-Dempsey & Sandler, 1997, p. 17). Rather than focusing on the types of activities parents engage in, self-efficacy captures parents' beliefs about how their activities affect their child's school competencies. Similar to findings on role construction, research has consistently linked self-efficacy beliefs to parents' involvement practices (Hoover-Dempsey *et al.*, 1992; Grolnick *et al.*, 1997; Hoover-Dempsey & Sandler, 1997).

We extend the research on connections between parent beliefs and involvement practices in a couple of important ways. First, we examine the connection between beliefs and practice among an understudied population, low-income rural fathers. Second, we study the relationship between a multiple-risk factors view of barriers to involvement, father beliefs and father involvement. If, as suggested by the literature, beliefs are most proximal to behaviors, we would expect pro-involvement beliefs to compensate for barriers. That is, fathers who consider it their role to be involved in their child's education and believe they can contribute through their behaviors may be more willing to push past obstacles to involvement. We test this premise by examining fathers' sense of self-efficacy and parental role construction (Hoover-Dempsey & Sandler, 1997) as mediators between contextual barriers and involvement behaviors.

Methods

Procedures

This study includes fathers and father figures of children enrolled in a HS or EHS intervention program in the Midwestern USA. There are 12 sites that serve approximately 225 children in a 4-county area each program year. All children enrolled met the admission guidelines based on poverty or disability status. Fathers who were identified on enrollment applications were invited to participate. In cases where fathers were not identified, mothers were asked to name the child's father or father figure, if applicable. Questionnaires and informed consent forms were sent to fathers, along with the following instructions:

> You have been given this survey because you are a father or a father figure to a child enrolled in a Head Start or Early Head Start program. This survey will be used to help us better understand the role that fathers or father figures play in the education of children. The information is anonymous in that your name is not linked to any information that you provide. If you have more than one child in the program, choose one child for the purposes of this survey. Answer the rest of the survey questions in the relation to the child that you choose.

Surveys were returned in sealed envelopes to the child's teacher or family advocate.

Participants

The sample included 101 fathers of infants and preschoolers (52% males, 48% females) between the ages of one and five. Approximately, 20% of the children were enrolled in EHS (age zero to three), while the remainder were enrolled in HS (age three to five). Seventy-five percent of participants were biological fathers, 5% were stepfathers, 6% were cohabitating partners, 4% were boyfriends not living with the mother, and 10% were relatives (uncles or grandfathers). Fathers and father figures will be referred to as fathers from this point on. Fathers reported that the majority of children had lived most of their life with both married parents (67%), while the remainder lived with: both married parents until divorce (4%), with his/her mother (22%), with his/her father (1%), with other relatives (2%), with his/her adoptive parents (1%), or in other living arrangements (3%). All fathers reported living with the child at least one day per week at the time of the study. Eighty percent of fathers were White, 6% Asian-American, 5% Native American, 1% African-American, 1% Hispanic, and 7% reported 'other' ethnicities. Fathers' age varied within the following categories: Younger than 20 (1%), 20–30 (25%), 30–40 (42%), 40–50 (26%), 50–60 (4%), and older than 60 (2%). Participants' educational backgrounds also varied considerably: some or completed high school (50%), some college (31%), a four-year degree (10%), and graduate or professional degree (8%).

Measures

Fathering context. Demographic variables were included as a measure of fathering context. Fathers were asked 'What is your relationship to the child?' Response choices included: biological father, stepfather, living with child's mother, boyfriend to child's mother (not living in child's house), grandfather, uncle, older brother, family friend, cousin, or other. This variable was re-coded into biological father or non-biological father figure. Father age was measured using a five-point response scale including: <20, 20–30, 30–40, 40–50, and >50 years old.

Perceived barriers to involvement were measured by asking fathers to rate responses to the following stem: 'I don't get to do all of the things that I like to with this child because of …' Six responses were rated on a five-point Likert response scale ranging from 1 = 'disagree' to 5 = 'agree,' and included: (1) lack of time, (2) energy, (3) resources/money, (4) work schedules or responsibilities, (5) stress, and (6) the child's mother prefers to be more involved with the child. Green *et al.* (2007) suggest that in particular, time and energy need to be examined together in relation to parental role and efficacy beliefs as they influence involvement. In order to measure the total impact of perceived barriers, each barrier was coded as 'perceived' (father rating of 4–5) or 'not-perceived' (father rating of 1–3). The total of perceived barriers, renamed as multiple risk factors, was calculated by summing the perceived barriers; a total multiple risk factor score ranged from 0–6.

Father role construction and efficacy. Father beliefs were measured using three scales that aligned with Hoover-Dempsey and Sandler's (1995, 1997) model of parent involvement (Green *et al.* 2007) and Lamb's model of father involvement (Lamb *et al.*, 1987). Measured constructs included: father efficacy, father role activity beliefs, and father responsibility to the intervention program. Average scores were computed across items for each scale. The *Father efficacy subscale* was measured using 11 items assessing fathers' perceived ability to help the child grow, develop, and learn (alpha = .73). This scale was adapted from Hoover-Dempsey *et al.*'s (1992) Parent Perceptions of Parent Efficacy Scale; items were reworded to address development and learning in the preschool period, as opposed to the school-age period; sample questions include: 'My efforts to help my child learn are successful' and 'I know how to help my child do well in preschool/childcare.' Items were rated on a five-point response scale from 0 = 'not at all' to 4 = 'very much,' and negatively worded items were re-coded. The *Father role activity beliefs subscale* measured fathers' beliefs about their role in the target child's development and education (see Hoover-Dempsey & Sandler, 1995; Hoover-Dempsey *et al.* 2005; Green *et al.* 2007). The four items assessed components of fathers' role including: making sure the child attends and is prepared for preschool or intervention activities, and talking with the teacher about things that concern the child. Fathers rated how strongly they agreed with role statements using a four-point Likert-type response scale from 0 = 'not at all' to 4 = 'very much' (alpha = .70). The *Father responsibility to the intervention program subscale* included four reverse-worded items that measured fathers' feelings of responsibility for the child's learning and interactions with the child's teacher or family advocate. These items were also rated on a four-point response scale from 0 = 'not at all' to 4 = 'very much.' Sample items included: 'I assume my child is doing all right if I don't hear anything from his or her teachers' and 'My child's learning is up to the teacher and my child' (alpha = .62).

Father involvement.   Father involvement was measured using an adapted version of the engagement items in the national Early Head Start Research and Evaluation Project (see Cabrera *et al.*, 2004), and was additionally based on Hoover-Dempsey and Sandler's (2005) constructs of home and school involvement (see Green *et al.* 2007). Four father involvement subscales were computed from items measuring four types of involvement: (1) *physical play*, (2) *didactic engagement*, (3) *caregiving*, and (4) *socialization* (Cabrera *et al.*, 2004). For the items measuring fathers' physical play and didactic interactions, fathers were asked: 'How many times per week do you get a chance to do each of the following activities with your preschool child?' Respondents rated the response choices on a six-point scale ranging from 1 = ' rarely' to 6 = '5+ times per week.' *Physical play* was computed by averaging fathers' level of involvement on 10 physical, exploratory, or active play items, including: playing pretend games, playing outdoor games, playing blocks, playing with sand, water, dirt, or snow, helping the child with large motor activities such as bikes or slides, rough housing with the child, building or fixing something together (real or pretend), doing art activities together, dancing together, and teasing or joking with the child to get him/her to laugh (alpha = .88). *Didactic play* was computed by averaging fathers' level of involvement on eight interactive, mentoring, or instructional play items, including: singing, telling, or reading nursery rhymes or books, telling or listening to stories with child, playing sharing games, playing with puppets, and playing computer games with the child (alpha = .82).

For the items measuring caregiving and socialisation, fathers were asked: 'Please rate how frequently you (not your spouse or partner) participate in each of these activities with your child.' Respondents 1 rated 17 response choices on a five-point scale ranging from 0 = 'never' to 4 = 'always.' *Caregiving* was computed by averaging fathers' responses to 10 items representing caregiving in the home including: eating with the child, supervising the child's bathing/teeth-brushing, talking and playing with the child, caring for the child during non-work hours or when the child is sick, washing the child's clothing and helping the child clean his/her room, letting the child 'help' at home (cooking, yardwork, etc.) and engaging in a bedtime routine with the child (alpha = .89). *Socialisation* was computed by averaging fathers' level of involvement on seven items measuring activities that engage the child in public settings or with other people outside of the immediate family including: taking the child to a birthday party or friend's house, the grocery store, library, dentist or doctor, to other activities, to buy clothes, and on outings (zoo, restaurant, etc.) (alpha = .83).

Father involvement in the program was measured with four items rated on a five-point scale ranging from 0 = 'never' to 4 = 'frequently.' Fathers were asked to rate how often they were involved in activities related to HS/EHS including: looking at their child's work (from school or home visits), keeping an eye on the child's progress, and exchanging notes or getting advice from the child's teacher or family advocate (alpha = .79). This scale most closely aligns with Hoovers-Dempsey *et al.*'s (2005) notion of school involvement, although the items reflect the type of involvement typical of an early childhood intervention program as opposed to a school setting.

Additionally, an accessibility score was used as an indicator of father involvement. In contrast to past research, in this study every father reported living with the child at least one day per week. Thus, residential status was not an adequate measure of father accessibility but rather reflected the fathering context. Instead, frequency of father contact was used as an indication of *accessibility to the father* (see Cabrera *et al.*, 2004). Fathers were asked 'On average, how many hours a week are you with this child,' and rated this item on a six-point scale ranging from 1 = 'less than 5' to 6 = 'greater than 35.'

Data analysis plan

Fathers' beliefs were examined as a mediator between fathering context and father involvement, following the procedures described by Barron and Kenny (1986). Pearson correlation and multiple regression analyses were conducted to test the following relationships: (1) associations between fathering context (i.e. multiple risk factors, biological status, father age) and mediating variables (i.e. father efficacy, role activity beliefs, and responsibility to the program), (2) prediction from fathering context to the dependent variables (father involvement), and (3) prediction from fathering context to involvement, controlling for the mediating variables. In a perfect mediating model 'the independent variable has no effect when the mediator is controlled' (Barron & Kenny, 1986, p. 1177).

Descriptive statistics

Context variables.   Descriptive statistics and intercorrelations for key study variables are presented in Table 1. Seventy-five percent of the fathers in this study were biological fathers (75%), while 25% were non-biological father figures. The most frequent age reported was 30–40 years old (42%), the next most frequent age reported was 20–30 and 40–50 years old (25% and 26% respectively) A few fathers fell in the lowest (<20) and highest (>50) ages ranges (1% and 6% respectively). On average, fathers agreed that three of the six risk factors inhibited their involvement with their child. Eighty percent of fathers perceived time and work schedules as barriers, while approximately 50% perceived lack of energy and resources as barriers, and approximately 33% reported stress and maternal gate-keeping as barriers to father involvement.

Father beliefs.   On average, fathers somewhat agreed with efficacy statements, although there was quite a bit of variability in their responses. Fathers tended to agree with the role activity belief statements, but were less likely to agree with the responsibility to the invention program statements (average responses were closer to 'disagree' than 'agree').

Father involvement.   The majority of fathers reported greater involvement in physical play activities (average was two to three times per week) compared with didactic play activities (average was two times per week). For caregiving and socialisation variables, fathers reported engaging in caregiving activities more frequently (average response was 'often') than socialisation activities (average responses were 'rarely' and 'sometimes'). Most fathers reported program involvement as 'occasionally' and 'sometimes.' Lastly, fathers reported considerably variability in being accessible (average response was 25–35 hours per week, but ranged from less than 5 hours to over 35 hours per week).

Correlation coefficients

Table 1 shows the correlations between fathering context and fathering beliefs. Biological status was not related to father beliefs, but father age and risk factors were inversely related to efficacy. Biological status generally showed a positive, but non-significant relationship with father involvement. Both father age and number of risk factors were negatively and statistically significantly associated with father involvement variables, except for the associations between father age with accessibility and program involvement.

Table 1 also shows small to moderate, positive correlations between father beliefs and father involvement across all measures of father involvement. Father

Table 1. Descriptive statistics and correlations

Father variable	Mean	SD	Range	Fathering context			Father beliefs			Father involvement					
				1	2	3	4	5	6	7	8	9	10	11	12
1. Biological status	—[a]	—	—	—	.05	-.12	.05	.08	-.10	.01	-.02	.14	.11	.09	.11
2. Father age	—[a]	—	—	—	—	-.04	-.20*	-.17	-.13	-.33***	-.34***	-.28**	-.36**	-.12	.02
3. Risk factors	3.12	1.58	0.00–6.00	—	—	—	-.30**	-.18	.02	-.20*	-.18	-.22*	-.22*	-.29**	-.23*
4. Efficacy	3.33	.54	2.00–4.56	—	—	—	—	.29**	.18	.43***	.46**	.38***	.32***	.30***	.23*
5. Role activity beliefs	3.10	.61	1.50–4.00	—	—	—	—	—	.19	.32***	.28**	.56***	.52***	.60***	.45**
6. Responsibility to program	2.41	.61	1.00–4.00	—	—	—	—	—	—	.06	-.07	.15	-.03	.14	.04
7. Physical play	3.34	1.14	1.11–6.00	—	—	—	—	—	—	—	.81**	.67***	.57***	.51**	.39**
8. Didactic play	3.07	1.11	1.00–6.00	—	—	—	—	—	—	—	—	.57***	.51***	.47**	.32**
9. Caregiving	3.58	.83	1.33–5.00	—	—	—	—	—	—	—	—	—	.78***	.56**	.52**
10. Socialisation	2.89	.81	1.00–5.00	—	—	—	—	—	—	—	—	—	—	.51**	.41**
11. Program involvement	3.24	1.01	1.00–5.00	—	—	—	—	—	—	—	—	—	—	—	.42**
12. Accessibility	—[a]	—	—	—	—	—	—	—	—	—	—	—	—	—	—

[a]Descriptive statistics for these variables are found in the text.
*p < .05, **p < .01.

efficacy and role construction were consistently related to father involvement with generally moderate to strong, positive, and statistically significant associations. The weakest associations were between father responsibility and father involvement. All father involvement variables were moderately to strongly, positively intercorrelated. Interestingly, fathers' involvement in EHS and HS programs was moderately and positively correlated with the two play variables, caregiving, socialisation, and accessibility to the child.

Regression analyses

Table 2 shows a series of regressions that were run to test the effect of contextual variables on father involvement variables (Step 1), and the effects of contextual variables when controlling for father belief variables (Step 2). Each of the regression models was statistically significant. In each model, contextual variables significantly predict father involvement variables in Step 1. However, in Step 2, contextual risk factors dropped out as a significant predictor of all types of involvement when father beliefs (i.e. fathers' efficacy, role activity beliefs, and responsibility to the program) were added into the models. The exception was for father age, which remained a significant unique predictor of father physical and didactic play, caregiving, and socialisation.

The R^2 or shared variability between the predictor variables and the dependent variables for each model doubled in Step 2 as a result of adding in father efficacy, role beliefs, and responsibility to program variables, which were significant unique predictors of involvement across all models. Specific types of beliefs predicted specific types of involvement, as shown in Table 2. For the dependent variables physical and didactic play, father efficacy mediated the influence of contextual variables. For caregiving, all three father belief variables significantly mediated the influence of contextual variables. For socialisation, involvement in the program, and accessibility, father role beliefs were a significant mediator of contextual variables.

Discussion

Taken together the findings offer compelling evidence for the hypothesis that father beliefs function as a mediator between family context and father involvement. Consistent with previous studies, a negative association was found between contextual barriers and parent involvement. In the current study we collapsed individual barriers into a multiple risk factor scale and results indicated that as the number of barriers increased fathers reported less socialisation, physical play, caregiving, program involvement, and accessibility. When father efficacy and role construction were taken into account; however, barriers no longer predicted father involvement. In a series of six hierarchical regressions examining the joint contributions of barriers and beliefs to six father involvement variables the results were consistent; beliefs mediated barriers in every case. According to Barron and Kenny (1986), a good measure of a mediator's potency is noting the degree to which its inclusion in the

Table 2.   Regression analyses predicting father involvement from fathering context and father beliefs

Variables entered	B	SEB	β	R^2	Adj. R^2
Dependent variable: Physical play				.15**	.12
Predictors Step 1					
Biological status	.07	.27	.02		
Father age	−.41	.12	−.33**		
Risk factors	−.17	.07	−.22*		
Predictors Step 2				.31***	.25
Biological status	.07	.26	.02		
Father age	−.31	.12	−.25**		
Risk factors	−.05	.07	−.06		
Efficacy	.80	.22	.38***		
Role activity beliefs	.20	.20	.10		
Responsibility to program	.29	.19	.15		
Dependent variable: Didactic play				.16**	.13
Predictors Step 1					
Biological status	.06	.27	.02		
Father age	−.43	.12	−.35***		
Risk factors	−.14	.07	−.19*		
Predictors Step 2				.34***	.29
Biological status	−.05	.25	−.02		
Father age	−.33	.11	−.27**		
Risk factors	−.02	.07	−.03		
Efficacy	.88	.21	.42***		
Role activity beliefs	.15	.19	.08		
Responsibility to program	.37	.18	.20*		
Dependent variable: Caregiving				.14**	.11
Predictors Step 1					
Biological status	.17	.19	.09		
Father age	−.24	.08	−.27**		
Risk factors	−.12	.05	−.23*		
Predictors Step 2				.42***	.7
Biological status	.09	.16	.04		
Father age	−.16	.07	−.18*		
Risk factors	−.03	.04	−.05		
Efficacy	.39	.14	.27**		
Role activity beliefs	.53	.12	.39***		
Responsibility to program	.24	.12	.18*		
Dependent variable: Socialisation				.16**	.13
Predictors Step 1					
Biological status	.14	.18	07		
Father age	−.29	.08	−.34***		
Risk factors	−10	.05	−.20*		
Predictors Step 2				.36***	.3
Biological status	.08	.16	.04		

Table 2.   *(Continued)*

Variables entered	B	SEB	β	R^2	Adj. R^2
Father age	−.21	.08	−.26**		
Risk factors	−.03	.05	−.06		
Efficacy	.22	.14	.16		
Role activity beliefs	53	.12	40***		
Responsibility to program	.03	.12	.02		
Dependent variable: Involvement in program				.10*	.06
Predictors Step 1					
Biological status	06	27	.02		
Father age	−.16	.12	−.14		
Risk factors	−.20	.07	−.28**		
Predictors Step 2				.42***	.37
Biological status	.09	.23	.04		
Father age	−.07	.11	−.06		
Risk factors	−.09	.06	−.13		
Efficacy	.25	.20	.13		
Role activity beliefs	.98	.17	.53***		
Responsibility to program	.13	.16	.07		
Dependent variable: Accessibility				.08*	.05
Predictors Step 1					
Biological status	.30	.30	.11		
Father age	.01	.14	.01		
Risk factors	−.17	.08	−.22*		
Predictors Step 2				.21**	.15
Biological status	.24	.29	.08		
Father age	.11	.13	.08		
Risk factors	−.08	.08	−.10		
Efficacy	.31	.25	.14		
Role activity beliefs	.67	.22	.33**		
Responsibility to program	.02	.2	.01		

$*p < .05; **p < .01; ***p < .001.$

model reduces the association between the predictor variable and the criterion. In this study, accounting for father efficacy and beliefs decreased the association between perceived barriers and fathers' involvement by one-half to a sixth of the zero order correlation.

The finding that personal beliefs trump physical circumstances or challenges is embodied in Western cultures' most cherished ideal; that individuals can accomplish what they put their minds to, despite the limitations imposed by personal background or their current situation. Examples of this belief can be found in the success of self-help books selling personal affirmations (i.e. 'I am beautiful, intelligent and lovable'), or in children's stories such as *The little engine that could* (Piper, 1961) a simple but inspiring tale of how believing in one's ability is enough to overcome seemingly impossible barriers. Like the story, Hoover-Dempsey and Sandler's model places parents' beliefs as the engine that drives behaviour, independent of social class, geography, cultural background, or even skills and knowledge (Green *et al.*, 2007). But unlike the children's story, the science of behavior clearly shows that the quality and quantity of parent–child interaction are not context free and that parent beliefs are not formed in a vacuum. Living below the poverty line, and especially chronic economic deprivation, has clear negative consequences on childrearing practices (McLoyd, 1998). In addition, social context plays a powerful role in shaping parents' perceptions of their capacity to influence the course of their child's education and development (Hoover-Dempsey *et al.*, 2005).

Barron and Kenny (1986) state that 'mediators explain how external physical events take on internal psychological significance' (p. 1176). Applying this to father involvement, research suggests social contexts become internalised as beliefs that motivate parents to engage their child in play, provide care, or other socialisation experiences. While our study shows how internalised beliefs mediate the association between context and behavior, it does little to explain correlates or origins of father beliefs. The number of perceived barriers was negatively associated with all three father belief variables, but only father efficacy reached a level of statistical significance. While the weak effect sizes of the bivariate correlations are consistent with other studies examining connections between barriers and beliefs (see Green *et al.*, 2007), they leave the majority of variance unaccounted for. Obviously other contextual influences, as well as personality factors, must play a significant role in shaping father's perceptions of their role and responsibility to their child's education. Hoover-Dempsey *et al.* (2005) also discuss the role of context as a direct influence, which limits or enhances involvement options.

HS and EHS are national efforts to create a positive social context for father involvement. A good measure of the success of HS and EHS is the degree to which parent involvement increases. But perhaps a better measure is the degree to which parents' successful involvement experiences are associated with positive gains in beliefs, including self-efficacy and positive paternal and maternal role construction. In fact, increased participation without a change in beliefs is unlikely to sustain parent's involvement practices or lead to greater parenting satisfaction (Fagan & Stevenson, 2002) once HS and EHS active recruiting of parent participation ends. Alternatively, if parents internalise new roles and beliefs about their ability to influence their child's academic success based on their experiences in HS, they are more likely to continue their involvement practices after their transition out of the program. Currently, predicting later behaviour from beliefs remains speculative and awaits longitudinal data that can follow families beyond HS.

A closer examination of the associations between context, beliefs, and behavior variables reveals a nuanced pattern of relationships. Father efficacy predicted higher involvement in physical and didactic play, and caregiving but not socialisation, program involvement or accessibility. In contrast, role construction was positively associated with all behavior outcomes except the two play behaviours, didactic and physical. Fathers' perceived responsibility to the program was the least predictive of the three belief variables, revealing only weak associations with didactic play and caregiving behaviour. This variable had weaker internal consistency that likely restricted associations with other variables in the study. Given that role construction was the most robust indicator of father behaviours, it is important to consider the social and cultural context that shapes fathers sense of personal responsibility for their child's education and development (Brannen & Nilsen, 2006).

Cultural and economic conditions in the developed world have propelled fathers into the childrearing spotlight, whether by personal choice or economic necessity (Pleck, 1987). Studies in Europe and the USA have documented a generational shift from the predominant 'breadwinner' role of the 1950s to today's father who is more apt to participate in daily childcare activities such as changing diapers, scheduling daycare arrangements[1], assisting with homework and meeting with teachers (Brannen & Nilsen, 2006). Still, it remains less clear if such cultural shifts in father involvement reflect concomitant changes in fathers' personal beliefs regarding their role in their child's caretaking and schooling (Eggebeen & Knoester, 2001). In some cases, household observations have shown that when both parents are available to the child, fathers do not engage in childrearing activities to a greater extent than males of previous generations (O'Brien & Shemilt, 2003). Active or 'rough and tumble' play, companionship, and shared activities are still the predominate modes of father–child interaction, whereas father initiated caretaking is rarely observed (see Newland, Coyl, and Freeman in this volume for a more complete review of this research). In other words, it may be that fathers become involved in childrearing practices and their child's education to the extent that it is demanded of them or to the extent that their family context or child's school necessitates or limits their involvement, but their beliefs concerning their role and efficacy may not be consistent with these activities. The current findings reveal a considerable range in father beliefs regarding their role and responsibility to their child's program and academic success, and show a consistent association between role beliefs and behaviour. As Hoover-Dempsey has suggested, the relationship between beliefs and behavior is likely bidirectional, such that father beliefs motivate fathers to become involved, which, in turn, reinforces their beliefs. Although this recursive relationship is likely to be moderated by other factors such as the fathers' satisfaction with their participation and opportunities for continued interactions. Longitudinal data would be necessary to tease apart the bi-directional nature and changes in these variables over time.

In the current study, the use of single source data may have contributed to shared method variance and overrepresented the connection between beliefs and behaviors, such that fathers' perceptions of barriers overlapped with their ratings of involvement and efficacy. Further work in this area would benefit from using an objective assessment of barriers where possible, such as documenting work schedules, hours available to child, and daily stressors.

Study findings support previous work suggesting that empowerment based interventions show greater promise than skill- or knowledge-based programs by themselves. An empowerment practice approach that acknowledges fathers' strengths and abilities, while enhancing parenting skills and knowledge of child development has been implemented in some early intervention programs. One example of this self-help approach is the *Men as Teachers* program designed for African-American fathers. A primary objective of the program is to improve fathers' parenting attitudes and parenting satisfaction. Actual participating HS fathers were recruited, helped develop, and were trained to deliver the program to other HS fathers. Results indicated a significant improvement in resident fathers' attitudes about their abilities to teach preschool children and reported a greater sense of self-esteem and parenting satisfaction but not among non-resident fathers (Fagan & Stevenson, 1995). Changing beliefs by building on what fathers already know and can do is likely to be a more sustainable road to father involvement. In closing we provide a few inspirational words from the *Little Engine that Could*:

> To think of hard things and say, 'I can't' is sure to mean 'Nothing done.' To refuse to be daunted and insist on saying, 'I think I can,' is to make sure of being able to say triumphantly by and by, 'I thought I could, I thought I could.'

Acknowledgements

The authors wish to thank the families and staff at USD Head Start Pre-Birth through Five. Their participation and assistance were invaluable. Data for this manuscript were derived from a larger study of father involvement funded through a Special Fatherhood Initiative Grant awarded to Head Start Pre-Birth through Five at USD through The Administration on Children, Youth and Families grant # ACYF-IM-HS-02-06. We also wish to thank Rita Humphrey for her assistance with manuscript preparation and revision.

Note

1. Recently when the first-author was immersed in thinking about cultural and socioeconomic shifts in fathering he was picking up his children from an in-home rural daycare and noticed that his arrival often coincided with that of three other fathers, but no mothers. Beyond using the same daycare the fathers shared little in common; the author being 20 years older than the youngest father and the only professional among two farmers and a mechanic. Although this personal observation may or may not be representative, it is perhaps more telling that this daily event went unnoticed until he began writing a paper about it.

References

Allen, S. M. & Hawkins, A. J. (1999) Maternal gatekeeping: mothers' beliefs and behaviors that inhibit greater father involvement in family work, *Journal of Marriage and the Family*, 61, 199–212.

Amato, P. R. & Gilbreth, J. G. (1999) Nonresident fathers and children's well-being: a meta-analysis, *Journal of Marriage & Family*, 61(2), 557–573.

Amato, P. R. & Rivera, F. (1999) Paternal involvement and children's behavior problems, *Journal of Marriage and Family*, 61(2), 375–384.

Barron, R. M. & Kenny, D. A. (1986) The moderator-mediator variable distinction in social psychological research: conceptual, strategic, and statistical considerations, *Journal of Personality and Social Psychology*, 51(6), 1173–1182.

Beitel, A. H. & Parke, R. D. (1998) Paternal involvement in infancy: the role of maternal and paternal attitudes, *Journal of Family Psychology*, 12, 268–288.

Boller, K., Bradley, R., Cabrera, N. *et al.* (2006) The Early Head Start father studies: design, data collection, and summary of father presence in the lives of infants and toddlers, *Parenting: Science and Practice*, 6(2), 117–143.

Brannen, J. & Nilsen, A. (2006) From fatherhood to fathering: transmission and change among British fathers in four-generation families, *Sociology*, 40(2), 335–352.

Brotman, L. M., Klein, R. G., Kamboukos, D., Brown, E. J., Coard, S. I. & Sosinsky, L. S. (2003) Preventive intervention for urban, low-income preschoolers at familial risk for conduct problems: a randomized pilot study, *Journal of Clinical Child and Adolescent Psychology*, 32(2), 246–257.

Bruce, C. & Fox, G. L. (1999) Accounting for patterns of father involvement: age of child, father–child coresidence, and father role salience, *Sociological Inquiry*, 69, 458–476.

Cabrera, N. J., Shannon, J. D., Vogel, C. *et al.* (2004) Low-income fathers' involvement in their toddlers' lives: biological fathers from the Early Head Start research and evaluation study, *Fathering*, 2, 5–30.

Cabrera, N. J., Tamis-LeMonda, C., Bradley, R. H., Hofferth, S. & Lamb, M. E. (2000) Fatherhood in the twenty-first century, *Child Development*, 71, 127–136.

Coleman, J. S. (1991) A federal report on parental involvement in education, *Education Digest*, 57(3), 3–6.

Collignon, F. F., Men, M. & Tan, S. (2001) Finding was in: community-based perspectives on southeast Asian family involvement with schools in a New England state, *Journal of Education for Students Placed at Risk*, 6(1, 2), 27–44.

Eggebeen, D. J. & Knoester, C. (2001) Does fatherhood matter for men? *Journal of Marriage and Family*, 63, 381–393.

Epstein, J. L. (1991) Effects on student achievement of teachers' practices of parent involvement, in: S. Silvern (Ed.) *Advances in reading/language research: Vol. 5. Literacy through family, community, and school interaction* (Greenwich, CT, JAI), 261–276.

Fagan, J. & Iglesias, A. (1999) Father involvement program effects on fathers, father figures, and their Head Start children: a quasi-experimental study, *Early Childhood Research Quarterly*, 14, 243–269.

Fagan, J. & Stevenson, H. (1995) Men as teachers: a self-help program on parenting for African American men, *Social Work with Groups*, 17(4), 29–42.

Fagan, J. & Stevenson, H. C. (2002) An experimental study of an empowerment-based intervention for African American Head Start fathers, *Family Relations*, 51, 191–198.

Garcia Coll, C., Akiba, D., Palacios, N. *et al.* (2002) Parental involvement in children's education: lessons from three immigrant groups, *Parenting: Science and Practice*, 2(3), 303–324.

Green, C. L., Walker, J. M. T., Hoover-Dempsey, K. V. & Sandler, H. M. (2007) Parents' motivations for involvement in children's education: an empirical test of a theoretical model of parental involvement, *Journal of Educational Psychology*, 99(3), 532–544.

Grolnick, W. S., Benjet, C., Kurowski, C. O. & Apostoleris, N. H. (1997) Predictors of parent involvement in children's schooling, *Journal of Educational Psychology*, 89(3), 538–548.

Grossman, F. K., Pollack, W. S. & Golding, E. (1988) Fathers and children: predicting the quality and quantity of fathering, *Developmental Psychology*, 24, 82–91.

Hess, R. D., Holloway, S. D., Dickson, W. P., Price, G. G. (1984) Maternal variables as predictors of children's school readiness and later achievement in vocabulary and mathematics in sixth grade, *Child Development*, 55(5), 1902–1912.

Hoover-Dempsey, K. V., Bassler, O. C. & Brissie, J. S. (1992) Explorations in parent-school relations, *Journal of Educational Research*, 85, 287–294.

Hoover-Dempsey, K. V. & Sandler, H. M. (1995) Parental involvement in children's education: why does it make a difference? *Teachers College Record*, 97, 310–331.

Hoover-Dempsey, K. V. & Sandler, H. M. (1997) Why do parents become involved in their children's education? *Review of Educational Research*, 67(1), 3–42.

Hoover-Dempsey, K. V., Walker, J. M., Sandler, H. M. *et al.* (2005) Why do parents become involved? Research findings and implications, *Elementary School Journal*, 106(2), 105–130.

Horvat, E. M., Weininger, E. B. & Lareau, A. (2003) From social ties to social capital: class differences in the relations between schools and parent networks, *American Educational Research Journal*, 40(2), 319–351.

Kellaghan, T., Sloane, K., Alvarez, B. & Bloom, B. (1993) *The home environment and school learning: promoting parental involvement in the education of children* (San Francisco, CA, Jossey-Bass).

King, V. (1994) Nonresident father involvement and child well-being: can dads make a difference? *Journal of Family Issues*, 15, 78–96.

King, V. & Heard, H. E. (1999) Nonresident father visitation, parental conflict, and mother's satisfaction: what's best for child well-being? *Journal of Marriage and the Family*, 61, 385–396.

Kissman, K. (2001) Interventions to strengthen noncustodial father involvement in the lives of their children, *Journal of Divorce and Remarriage*, 35(1/2), 135–146.

Lamb, M. E., Pleck, J. H., Charnov, E. L. & Levine, J. A. (1987) A biosocial perspective on paternal care and involvement, in: J. B. Lancaster, J. Altmann, A. Rossi & L. Sherrod (Eds.) *Parenting across the lifespan: biosocial perspectives* (Chicago, IL, Aldine), 111–142.

Lamb, M. E. (Ed.) (2004) *The role of the father in child development* (4th edn) (Hoboken, NJ, Wiley).

Madden-Derdich, D. A., Leonard, S. A. & Christopher, F. S. (1999) Boundary ambiguity and parental conflict after divorce: an empirical test of a family systems model of the divorce process, *Journal of Marriage and the Family*, 61, 588–598.

Matta, D. S. & Knudson-Martin, C. (2006) Responsivity: couple processes and the construction of fatherhood, *Family Processes*, 45, 19–37.

McBride, B., Brown, G., Bost, K., Shin, N., Vaughn, B. & Korth, B. (2005) Paternal identity, maternal gatekeeping, and father involvement, *Family Relations*, 54, 360–372.

McLoyd, V. C. (1998) Socioeconomic disadvantage and child development, *American Psychologist*, 53, 185–204.

O'Brien, M. & Shemilt, I. (2003) *Working fathers: earning and caring* (London, Equal Opportunities Commission).

Olson, S. L., Ceballo, R. & Park, C. (2002) Early problem behavior among children from low-income, mother-headed families: a multiple risk perspective, *Journal of Clinical Child and Adolescent Psychology*, 31(4), 419–430.

Piper, W. (1961) *The little engine that could.* (New York, Platt & Munk/Grosset & Dunlap).

Pleck, J. H. (1987) American fathering in historical perspective, in: M. S. Kimmel (Ed.) *Changing men: new directions in research on men and masculinity* (Newbury Park, CA, Sage).

Roggman, L. A., Boyce, L. K., Cook, G. A. & Cook, J. (2002) Getting dads involved: predictors of father involvement in Early Head Start and with their children, *Infant Mental Health Journal*, 23, 62–78.

Weiss, H. B., Mayer, E., Kreider, H. *et al.* (2003) Making it work: low-income working mothers' involvement in their children's education, *American Educational Research Journal*, 40(4), 879–901.

Fathers: the 'invisible' parents

Olivia N. Saracho[a] and Bernard Spodek[b]

[a]*University of Maryland, USA;* [b]*University of Illinois, USA*

The art of fatherhood is like all arts, long, tedious, exacting.

Angelo Patri,[1] 'Fathers.' (Radio script, 1932, cited in LaRossa, 1997, p. 144)

Introduction

Fathers are the family ghosts in relation to their children's development and well-being. Their contributions are too often merely attributed to the children's financial support. This pre-conceived notion has led researchers on child development to focus almost exclusively on mothers and their contributions to their children's lives. The few studies that have examined the fathers' involvement in the children's lives (Levine *et al.*, 1993) may have created the perception that fathers were the 'hidden parents.' Researchers need to gain insight into the norms, expectations, and beliefs that determine the fathers' involvement and what constitute culturally appropriate father–child activities. Such a research strand is indispensable in presenting an in-depth understanding of the fathers' roles as a result of their cultural factors, family's personal history, cultural beliefs, cultural values, language, and fathers' contributions to specific events. The purpose of this article is to discuss the measures and methodologies used to study father involvement. In addition, challenges to these studies will be discussed.

Historical patterns of fatherhood

Research studies on families have examined mother–child interactions, family systems, family general practices, or the mothers' family contributions. They have also ignored the fathers' multiple roles in the family. Father–child interactions were usually overlooked because researchers believed that the fathers' involvement was minimal and did not affect the children's development. As a result, studies have only reported on the absence or presence of fathers in the family environment. For example, Blankenhorn (1995) described how fathers were absent from family life as a result of changes in family structures (e.g., higher divorce rates, dramatically increased numbers of out-of-wedlock births, neglect). When fathers participated as equal family members, they often were characterised as being too busy elsewhere to be part of their children's learning. Durkin (1966), for example, made an effort to investigate the fathers' contributions to their young children's reading achievement. When she tried to interview the fathers, she received a number of excuses for interview refusals such as 'being on the road,' 'working during the day and going to school at night,' 'spending long hours at the office,' and 'having two jobs.' In addition, some fathers had difficulty establishing and maintaining positive and emotionally supportive relationships with their children due to their restricted resources, insecure employment, and lack of education (Cabrera *et al.*, 2004; Tamis-LeMonda *et al.*, 2004).

Contemporary social conditions have been progressively challenging fathers to assume an increasingly active role in child rearing. Unfortunately, many fathers have limited experience with children and lack the knowledge on how to assume the tasks and responsibilities of fatherhood. Fathers often state that they are ambiguous about their roles as fathers. In addition, they feel isolated from other fathers in relation to their paternal role (Fagan & Iglesias, 1999). Fathers who are economically challenged usually encounter many barriers to becoming involved with their children, including high rates of unemployment and joblessness, early childbearing outside of marriage, an unremitting succession of negative life events, and the absence of positive male role models (Furstenberg, 1995).

Sociodemographic, cultural, economic, and historical transformations, such as women's increased involvement in the labor force, the increase in non-parental care for children, the expansion in non-marital childbearing, increase in divorce, and the absence of fathers from their families have increased fathers' involvement in their children's lives, modifying the family's structure. The increase in fathers' involvement in their children's lives has contributed to the ways families are organizing themselves (Cabrera *et al.*, 2000). As a result of these transformations

- Fathers became the forerunners in the establishment of a variety of family structural systems, expectations, and beliefs concerning the roles of fathers and mothers.
- Fathers became the precursor for the diversity in family structures, expectations, and beliefs about the parental roles, suggesting that both mothers and fathers assumed and had overlapping family roles.
- Father ideals have evolved from the colonial father, to the distant breadwinner, to the modern involved father, to fathers as co-parents (Pleck & Pleck, 1997).

Lamb (2000) portrayed the evolution of fatherhood which shifted concepts about the major responsibility of the fathers. In his portrayal, fathers evolved from that of 'moral teacher or guide' before the Industrial Revolution to the role of 'breadwinner' that prevailed from the Industrial Revolution until the Great Depression. In the 1930s and 1940s, the 'sex-role model' emerged; while in the middle of the 1970s the 'new nurturant father' surfaced. Many have argued that culture defines the meaning of fatherhood. The evolution in culture changes standards in identifying effective or good fathers (Morman & Floyd, 2002).

Society has considered men to be good fathers when they provide their family with financial support; however, society has neglected to examine the quality of interactions between fathers and their children. Apparently, studies on this phenomenon are limited, but a sequence of changes has occurred. Scholars have analysed historical materials and have written about the past to help understand contemporary concerns and confusion about fatherhood. Pleck (1997) identified four themes over the last two centuries of American history.

(1) *Moral teacher or guide.* From the Puritan to the Colonial and into the early Republican periods, fathers were responsible for moral oversight and moral teaching. Good fathers were defined as men who assumed a model of good Christian living and helped their children become versed in the Scriptures.
(2) *Breadwinner.* From the mid-nineteenth century through the Great Depression, fatherhood was defined as breadwinning. Industrialization forced a separation between in- and out-of-home work. Breadwinning became the most important and defining characteristic of fatherhood. Good fathers were men who were breadwinners.
(3) *Sex-role model.* In the 1930s and early 1940s fathers continued to be breadwinners and moral guides; but their role was extended to become sex-role models, particularly to their sons. However, many believed that fathers were inadequate in this role and were ridiculed in dramatic works like *Rebel Without a Cause*, *Blondie*, and *All in the Family* (Ehrenreich & English, 1979).
(4) *New nurturant father.* The 1970s denoted a change in the importance of fatherhood. Fathers were defined as being nurturant parents who effectively participated in their children's daily care and this theme was used as a yardstick to determine who were 'good fathers.'

The aforementioned themes describe the complex roles that fathers have assumed throughout history. The literature on fathers makes it obvious that the term *father* refers to a multifaceted and diverse group of men in the families (Day & Lamb, 2004).

It is problematic to ignore the roles that fathers have assumed in their families. Marks and Palkovitz (2004) reported that the fathers' involvement had generally been taken for granted, had negative connotations, or were insufficiently conceptualised. For example, the extensive literature on the social features of fatherhood provided three broad dimensions of fatherhood: *fatherless and deadbeats, father–child interactions, and relationship between fathers and mothers*. The *fatherless and deadbeats* emphasized the implicit equation of responsible fatherhood with successful provisioning or breadwinning. Researchers who examined direct *father–child interactions* focused on the fathers' provision of care, discipline, coaching, education, companionship, play, and supervision. Studies on the *relationship between fathers and mothers* considered the family to be the most important determinant in the family context that contributed to the children's development and adjustment in important ways. Although the researchers focused on fatherhood, they failed to consider the interactions among the multiple roles and the ways in which a broader and more inclusive concept of fatherhood might both enrich and change the researchers' analysis and understanding. Biller (1974) purported that 'paternal deprivation, including patterns of inadequate fathering as well as father absence, is a highly significant factor in the development of serious psychological and social problems' (p. 1). He also made the case that, 'paternal deprivation is a term that can be used to include various inadequacies in a child's experience with his father' (p. 5). Hawkins and Dollahite (1997) characterized this belief to be the *deficit* model in the research on father, because this attitude focused mainly on the negative effects of father absence.

Research on father involvement

For about the past four decades, research on father involvement has multiplied (Cabrera *et al.*, 2004; Lamb, 2004; Tamis-LeMonda *et al.*, 2004). Early studies on father involvement only contrasted the absence or presence of fathers, their financial contributions, and the amount of time they spent with their children. More recent research has challenged their methodological and conceptual problems in these studies. Researchers then created multidisciplinary teams to restructure the scheme on fatherhood. These teams have altered how researchers conceptualised, collected, and measured data on fathers. They designed fresh research investigations that precisely conceptualised and measured father involvement as well as the effects that fathers' involvement had in their children's well-being and development. They disregarded the original belief that fathers failed to have an impact on the children's development and learning. During the earlier period, studies focused on the negative effects of the fathers' absence; whereas family studies usually focused on the mothers' contributions.

The family's traditional roles and responsibilities have been radically altered. The primary unit of mother and child dyad has been reconceptualized to include the importance of fathers, which has extended the concept of the American family structure. The studies on fathers extended their role, which has helped them to develop a father role identity and gain an understanding of the meaning of what it is to be a father (LaRossa, 1997; LaRossa & Reitzes, 1993). Paternity and economic demands have continuously been essential elements in good fathering; however, a contemporary model of 'co-parent' has emerged where the gender separation of work in household and financial responsibilities is eliminated (Pleck & Pleck, 1997). Family roles and responsibilities are gender-free. Both fathers and mothers have become co-parents where they equally share household, financial, and caregiving responsibilities.

Several researchers have been attempting to rebalance the family structure to give appropriate credit to the fathers' contributions. They have focused their attention on the fathers' involvement with their children as a result of the modifications in the women's work patterns and the men's personal interest in undertaking child care (Gerson, 1993; Parke, 1996). For example, Lamb (2004) reported that fathers, like mothers, are sensitive and responsive in their interactions with their young children. Donate-Bartfield and Passman (1985) found in their longitudinal study that the increased caretaking experience of the fathers has increased their responsiveness to their young children.

Current research studies support the concept that the fathers' involvement with their children affects their learning outcomes. The results from Nord *et al.*'s (1997) study showed that children usually achieved high marks, enjoyed school, and never repeated a grade when fathers of two-parent families engaged in school activities at a moderate or high level. The same results were found for those children whose fathers lived outside the home, but who also had a moderate or high level of school involvement in school. This study supports the contemporary perception that fathers have an important role in their children's learning and development.

The fathers' impact on their children's academic success has prompted a sequence of studies that investigated the nature, antecedents, and importance of the fathers' involvement with their children (Cabrera *et al.*, 2004; Shannon *et al.*, 2002; Tamis-LeMonda *et al.*, 2004). When fathers consistently encouraged and were involved with their children, their children achieved (1) better school performance (Nord *et al.*, 1997), (2) good self-esteem, (3) healthier relationships with peers, (4) healthier sex-role development (Green, 2003), (5) higher academic achievement (Nord *et al.*, 1997), and (6) better personal success.

Investigations examined how the fathers' involvement influenced their children's academic achievement, peer relationships, cognitive development, and behavioral or emotional regulation (Cabrera *et al.*, 2000; Tamis-LeMonda & Cabrera, 2002; Lamb, 2004). They showed that the fathers' involvement with their children, work environment, and cultural surroundings (Taylor & Behnke, 2005) modified their social roles (e.g., being a father) and behaviors in an effort to meet societal standards (Stryker & Statham, 1985). Ortiz and his colleagues (e.g., Ortiz *et al.*, 1999; Stile & Ortiz, 1999; Ortiz & Ordoñez-Jasis, 2005) recommended educational activities that would improve the quality of the father–child dyads. In a later study, Ortiz (2004) showed that the fathers' involvement affected their children's education; several themes emerged from their participation. These studies point out that fathers, like mothers, were responsible for their children, provided meaningful resources, and were meaning-makers in their children's family context.

Researchers also examined fathers' involvement in early childhood programs (Fagan, 2000; Lamb, 2004) in several domains: (1) the relationship between the children's developmental outcomes and patterns of the fathers' involvement and absence (e.g., Lamb, 2004); (2) the ways fathers balance economic provisions, household work, and participation in child-rearing practices (e.g., Palkovitz, 2002; Coltrane, 2004; Marks & Palkovitz, 2004); and (3) the relationship between the fathers' contributions and their children's literacy development (e.g., Ortiz, 2004; Saracho, 2007b), which has become of special interest. Durkin's (1966) study of young children's reading achievement showed that the few fathers who were interviewed seemed to have had a positive influence on their children's early reading achievement. Other researchers later supported these results. Saracho (2007b) reported the literacy experiences of fathers and their five-year-old children after a literacy intervention that was designed to assist fathers to foster their children's literacy development. She found that the fathers learned literacy strategies and activities that contributed to their children's acquisition of literacy. The literacy studies supported that the fathers could make important contributions to their children's literacy development.

Measurement approaches

Researchers who have examined the many facets of father involvement and their influence on child development have used various research designs and strategies. For more than two decades, scholars have explored work histories, economic fortunes, and fertility patterns of thousands of men. Later, researchers investigated the economic conditions, child care patterns, work histories, and payments to minor children. These studies are responding to important research questions about fathers and their families through systematic, careful, and small scale research designs based on ethnographic and qualitative methodologies. The research designs have provided opportunities to closely examine the subjects' individual behavior, motivation, and interpersonal interactions, providing more information than can be obtained from responses on survey questions. When researchers use a variety of research methods (both quantitative and qualitative) and research designs (e.g., experimental, quasi-experimental, survey, observations, interview), they are able to develop a comprehensive understanding of the fathers' role and influence within their families and children (Day & Lamb, 2004).

The shifting models of fatherhood have critically affected the kinds of activities, measures, and empirical methodologies to study father involvement. Since research evidence showed that the fathers' involvement has important implications for the family members, it is essential that fathers be considered an integral component of a family support system. It is important to consider contemporary methods that are used to measure father involvement and overcome all challenges in the process. To best understand the effects of father involvement on children's development, Cabrera *et al.* (2000) suggested that researchers consider (1) the specific *dimensions of father involvement*, (2) the *children's outcomes*, and (3) the *pathways* by which fathers influence their children.

Dimensions of father involvement

The unitary dimensions of father involvement need to be expanded to include broader and more inclusive definitions. For example, studies need to differentiate among *accessibility*, *engagement*, and *responsibility*. *Accessibility* considers the fathers' presence, interactions, and availability. *Engagement* includes the fathers' experience on direct contact, caregiving, and shared interactions with their children. *Responsibility* refers to how the fathers engage in duties like choosing a pediatrician and making appointments, deciding on child care settings or baby sitters, organising for after school child care and the care of sick children, discussing issues with teachers, and monitoring the children's whereabouts and activities (Lamb, 2004). Resident and non-resident fathers need to assume responsibility for financial child support. Co-resident parents need to assume managerial oversight and supervision. Characteristics of father–child interactions need to consider warmth, affection, sensitivity, and engagement in important aspects of the children's lives (Amato & Rejac, 1994).

Multiple dimensional structures of father involvement need to be integrated into a comprehensive theoretical framework. For example, the relationship among the different dimensions of father involvement and how changes in one dimension affect other dimensions. It is also important to consider the way father involvement functions (Parke & Buriel, 1997).

Children's outcomes.   Sociocultural situations require researchers to consider which patterns in the different dimensions of father involvement affect child development. The findings may be influenced by the dimensions of father involvement, type of fathers studied, and developmental stages and ages of the children. Researchers need to raise questions such as 'Which outcomes in children are most influenced by which dimensions of father involvement, at which developmental stages, and how?' (Cabrera *et al.*, 2000, p. 129). Initially the answers to these questions may have contradictory variations. There is little support that shows that the amount of father involvement provides desirable outcomes. For instance, fathers with financial means may spend less time with their children than fathers with a low income. However, their involvement has been found to be more positive (Levy-Shiff & Israelashvili, 1988). Similarly, when fathers lose their jobs and are forced into child care or parental duties while mothers keep their job, children do not profit; but they may suffer (Russell, 1983).

Influential pathways.   The family structure can be used to understand the fathers' *direct* and *indirect* influence on their children. The fathers' involvement with their children may *directly* affect child development similarly to the quality of mother–child attachment effects on child development. The fathers' ease of access may give their children a sense of security and emotional support. On the other hand, a harmonious family environment where subjects are happy may provide *indirect* effects in a study of the fathers' involvement (Lamb, 2004). Studies showed a relationship between marital harmony and the quality of parent–child relationships and their children's adjustment (Gable *et al.*, 1994); while marital conflict has been related to maladjustment (Cummings & O'Reilly, 1997).

Studies on the development of fatherhood are complicated by the fact that there is no singular set of developmental endpoints or tasks that define competent, supporting fathering for all men. Social trends (e.g., increased female employment, father absence, father involvement, cultural diversity) have influenced the transformations of the structures on the family environment and their expectations concerning the fathers' roles. The increased involvement of the fathers in child care suggested that they would assume more responsibility for child care and the foundation of their children's lives (Cabrera *et al.*, 2000).

Indices of father involvement

Studies have used several indices to assess father involvement. The major measurement methods to assess father involvement consisted of the use of time diaries, correlational studies that demonstrate the salience of father presence by studying families without fathers, and variations of Lamb *et al.*'s (1985) constructs of engagement, accessibility, and responsibility. According to Allen and Daly (2007), father involvement has typically been measured in one, or a combination, of the following three ways:

(1) *Time spent together* measured the frequency the fathers and children spent time together in activities such as in meals, during leisure time, play (i.e., effective, mutual, reciprocal), and reading. This method included the amount of time fathers engaged in routine physical child care (e.g., bathing, preparing meals, clothing).

(2) *Quality of the father–child relationship* measured the fathers' relationship (e.g., sensitive, warm, close, friendly, supportive, intimate, nurturing, affectionate, encouraging, comforting, accepting) and the children's extent of attachment to the father (like a strong and secure father–child attachment). However, Pleck (1997) believed that father involvement needs to distinguish between 'positive father involvement' (p. 67) and only 'father involvement' per se. Palkovitz (1997, 2000) suggested additional categories of paternal involvement:

  - Communication (listening, talking, showing love);
  - Teaching (role modeling, encouraging activities and interests);
  - Monitoring (friends, homework);
  - Cognitive processes (worrying, planning, praying);
  - Errands; Caregiving (feeding, bathing);
  - Shared interests (reading together);

- Availability;
- Planning (activities, birthdays);
- Shared activities (shopping, playing together);
- Providing (food, clothing);
- Affection; Protection; and
- Supporting emotionality (encouraging the child).

(3) *Investment in paternal role* measured the fathers' authoritative behavior management skills. Authoritative fathers used appropriate discipline, control, and limits; while simultaneously providing autonomy and monitoring of children's activities. This paternal role also included the fathers' ability to facilitate, be attentive to their children's needs, and to provide support to the children's school-related activities.

Research measurement challenges

For approximately four decades, the research on father involvement has increased (Cabrera *et al.*, 2004; Lamb, 2004; Tamis-LeMonda *et al.*, 2004). Although contemporary researchers have refined their methodologies, they continue to confront challenges and limitations in studies of fathers. The design of many studies continue to generate methodological and practical challenges when researchers make an effort to become knowledgeable about the nature and meaning of fathering (Cabrera *et al.*, 2004). Additionally, studies of fathers have raised methodological and conceptual debates in understanding fatherhood. Allen and Daly (2007) identified the following measurement challenges:

- *Multidimensional versus unidimensional conceptualisations* measured the relationship between father involvement and its different results. Since father involvement is a unidimensional construct, the fathers' direct involvement was assessed. However, many researchers argue that father involvement is complex and should be considered a 'multidimensional' construct (Schoppe-Sullivan *et al.*, 2004). Palkovitz (1997) includes 15 categories to defined father involvement (as described in the previous section). Parke (2000) maintained that the disposition of father involvement differs based on the children's developmental stages and the fathers' different developmental challenges. Fathers experience several transitions during their life (Palkovitz & Palm, 2005).
- *Environmental and other influences.* The fathers' involvement (e.g., activities, thoughts, engagements) with their children take place within a complex environment of other influences, which affects the quality and nature of any interactions. According to Palkovitz (2002):

> Because development is multiply determined and plastic, it is somewhat hazardous to get too specific regarding relationships between patterns of paternal involvement and child development outcomes. In focusing on child outcomes we often ignore the fact that patterns of father involvement are only one factor in a large and diverse array of possible contributors to developmental outcomes. The existing database does not allow us to conclusively partial out the effects of father involvement on child outcome variables. (p. 130)

Therefore, it is important that the results consider a wide range of influences on studying the fathers' involvement.

- *Measurement concerns.* Many studies have used questionable methodological procedures when examining the relationship between the fathers' involvement and their children's outcomes. Many researchers only use a single data source, with the same subjects providing the information on the fathers' involvement and their children's outcomes. In analysing the data, researchers usually depend on correlational and often cross-sectional computations. Therefore, these studies make it difficult to infer the direction of causality and to justify the selection effects or pre-existing conditions inherent in the children, thus challenging the results (Pleck & Masciadrelli, 2004).
- *Social economic status problems.* Often researchers have failed to control for social economic class in their studies of father involvement. Kesner and McKenry (2001) sustained that if studies in social skills and conflict management would control for socioeconomic class, no differences would be found between children from single- and two-parent families, indicating that a single parent family system may not be a risk factor in the children's social development (Kesner & McKenry, 2001). For example, Battle (2002) controlled for the family's socioeconomic status and did not find any statistical significance in predicting educational achievement.
- *Quality of child–parenting (mother and father) relationship.* When determining the effects of father involvement in the children's outcomes, researchers need to control for the effects that the child–mother relationship have on the children's outcomes and the quality of the fathers' child care. These factors could account for a portion of the observable effects. For example, Amato (1994) observed that the extent of the mothers' child care and the quality of the marriage may have accounted for the supposed positive effects of the fathers' child care. Rohner and Veneziano (2001) recommended that father involvement be investigated from a triadic (mother–father–child) or systemic standpoint instead of only examining a dyadic relationship (father–child).
- *Direct and indirect effects.* Most studies examine the direct effects of father involvement on child development outcomes; however, researchers need to consider how the fathers indirectly affect their children's developmental outcomes. When fathers provide mothers with practical and emotional support, the fathers improve the quality of the mother–child relationship, which affects the children's outcomes (Lamb, 2000). Also the fathers' accumulation of social capital, access to privilege, income, and social networks indirectly affect the children's outcomes.
- *Father presence and father absence effects.* The degree that the fathers are present in their children's lives may not affect the children's outcomes. For instance, fathers with antisocial behavior contribute to their children's behaviour problems (Jaffee *et al.*, 2003). Those who study men in families have taken a variety of approaches. At the end of World War II, a few child psychologists began to wonder about the effects of the men's long-term absence on the psychological well-being of their children. Stolz (1954) reported that some fathers were participants in World

War II and were absent at least during the first year following the birth of their children. This study represents an important conceptual starting point, because it is one of the few early studies in which fathers were not blamed for their absence. Unemployed father may be highly involved with their children; but since they prefer to be less involved to provide their children with financial support, they may have a negative contribution to the children's outcomes. Researchers suggest that the family context, family process, patterns of interaction, and the quality of various relationships are more important than father involvement (Davis & Friel, 2001). They believe that the fathers' presence or absence may not generate negative results on the children as would be factors such as (1) no co-parent, (2) economic loss/disadvantage, (3) social isolation and disapproval, (4) perceived/ actual abandonment relating to psychological distress, or (5) conflict between parents (Cabrera et al., 2000).

- *Fathers' employment conditions.* Some employment issues affect the fathers' involvement. For example, if fathers become unemployed and have to assume child care responsibilities, they may become harsh parents and have negative effects on them (Russell, 1983, cited in Allen & Daly, 2007). The fathers' involvement was influenced when families had employed or non-employed mothers. Fathers became more involved with their children when mothers worked (Lamb, 2000), when mothers earned more money than fathers (Casper & O'Connell, 1998), or when both parents have non-standard work schedules (Presser, 1995). On the other hand, fathers who earned a high income tended to become less involved with their children whereas fathers who earned a low income spent more positive time with their children (Levy-Shiff & Israelashvili, 1988).

Attempts to increase the quality of the fathers' involvement with their children have been the focus of some studies. Unfortunately, there are insufficient measures and indices of father involvement, which require the need of rigorous research tools. Measurement and strategies in fatherhood have focused on social problems (e.g., rates of unemployment, school drop out, teenage pregnancy, child support payment) instead of assessing the quality of fathering or the fathers' behaviour that affects their children's or family outcomes. Both conceptual and theoretical measures of father involvement are needed to examine the outcomes for fathers, families, and children. This requires a balanced and informed model that directly assesses fathers, fathering, and the fathers' contributions that improve the children's outcomes. This model needs to consider a range of possible problematic issues. Gadsden et al. (2004) suggested that the research model include (1) *defining the term 'father'*, (2) *using naive dichotomies*, (3) *constructing the fathers' roles as care givers*, (4) *capturing cultural variations*, and (5) *measuring the quantity versus quality of paternal involvement*.

(1) *Defining the term 'father'.* Many have used this term to refer to a biological father. Children may relate to different individuals who are assuming the role of a father, including biological fathers, stepfathers, mothers' partner, or male relatives who behave like a father. Studies that examine fathering need to identify ways to assess the roles of fathering when multiple individuals are involved.

(2) *Using naive dichotomies*. Fatherhood research that examine the fathers' contact, interactions, and responsibilities toward their children must factor in variables such as involved versus uninvolved father, intact versus father-absent homes, and financially contributing versus financially irresponsible fathers. Researchers can control these dichotomal representations of fatherhood. They can record a continuum of the fathers' involvement through multiple points of entry and exit and observe the nature of change in the children and their well being.

(3) *Constructing the fathers' roles as caregivers*. The fathers' roles as caregivers are difficult to assess. Researchers need to distinguish between the caregivers' roles of fathers and mothers to understand the fathers' and mothers' economic and caregiving contributions to the family. Researchers need to consider the development and evolutions of caregiving that are part of the fathers' identity, beliefs, and behaviors during the family's life course.

(4) *Capturing cultural variations*. Fathering indicators must be defined and refined in relation to cultures and communities determining which paternal roles are appropriate within a variety of cultural contexts. Values and beliefs may conflict with the researchers' perceptions of the father's role and those expected by specific cultures or communities. Differences among communities and cultures require that universal and flexible indicators be used with all groups. Studies need to acknowledge and incorporate the differences in fathering indicators among multiple cultures and communities. To be useful, fathering indicators need to be flexible so that they can easily be modified, expanded, rejected, or reshaped to reflect the specific culture and community that is being studied.

(5) *Measuring the quantity versus quality of paternal involvement*. Studies need to include both quantitative and qualitative measures of father involvement to obtain a comprehensive understanding of fatherhood (e.g., father–child interactions and its related underlying processes). For example, the nature and quality of father involvement can be collected along with the quantity of time spent in various activities and contexts.

Research studies continue to encounter challenges in studies of fatherhood, such as the lack of an accepted definition of fathers and fathering, a need for focused theoretical models concerning fathers, limited acknowledgment in the research literature on the cultural embeddedness and variability of fathering, obstacles in recruiting fathers to participate in research, and insufficient conceptual and theoretical measures to assess the fathers' involvement.

Conclusion

In general, studies of father involvement have various limitations that challenge our knowledge of father involvement and its consequences. Allen and Daly (2007) recommended that researchers consider measurement, sampling, and social class issues, to be attentive to direct and indirect effects, to consider the multidimensionality of father involvement within the context of other influences and relationships, to explore the impact of structural parameters on involvement such as employment conditions, and to find better ways of understanding father presence than by exploring its opposite—father absence. Studies that consider these limitations can contribute to research and theory on father involvement

Although contemporary researchers have refined their methodologies, researchers continue to confront challenges and limitations in studies of fathers. Although studies of fathers emerged, most research methods for studying mothers have been used in studies of father. In addition, studies have used mothers as the primary source of information about fathers. There is a need for methodological approaches that will provide accurate information by studying fathers directly or as members of a family. There have been many attempts to resolve the issues raised in researching fathers. Marks and Palkovitz (2004) proposed that the fathers' roles be conceptualised to provide an appropriate balance within the family structure. Researchers searched for an understanding of how fatherhood has been perceived and its transition from the traditional to the contemporary role of fathers.

Researchers need to evaluate their biases to avoid erroneous perceptions and misleading conceptions. They need to be sensitive and protect their studies from such assumptions and errors. They need to consider methodological and conceptual challenges to obtain an interpretive perspective and a better understanding of fathers' perceptions of other family members and the contributions and the general expectations that make up good fathering.

In addition, educators need to learn strategies to be able to make all family members feel comfortable in educational settings—fathers as well as mothers. Educational programs must assume the responsibility to reach out to all family members, especially to estranged ones. The possibility and responsibility of working with families, including fathers, demands that educators use the available wealth of home-based knowledge to inform their practice (Saracho, 2007a).

Note

1. Angelo Patri, a graduate of Columbia University (M.A. in Education), had a weekly radio show and syndicated newspaper column titled, 'Our Children.' He was well known for his books. He initiated his writing career with children's stories. He had a successful series on Pinocchio and later wrote several manuals on education and child-rearing practices.

References

Allen, S. & Daly, K. (2007) *The effects of father involvement: an updated research summary of the evidence.* Available online at: http://www.fira.ca/cms/documents/29/Effects_of_Father_Involvement.pdf (accessed 12 January 2008).

Amato, P. R. (1994) Father–child relationships, mother–child relations, and offspring psychological well-being in early adulthood, *Journal of Marriage and Family,* 56, 1031–1042.

Amato, P. R. & Rejac, S. J. (1994) Contact with non-resident parents, interparental conflict, and children's behavior, *Journal of Marriage and Family,* 15, 191–207.

Battle, J. (2002) Longitudinal analysis of academic achievement among a nationwide sample of Hispanic students in one- versus dual-parent households, *Hispanic Journal of Behavioral Sciences,* 24(4), 430–447.

Biller, H. B. (1974) *Paternal deprivation* (Lexington, MA, Heath).

Blankenhorn, D. (1995) *Fathers in America* (New York, Basic Books).

Cabrera, N., Ryan, R., Shannon, J., *et al.* (2004) Low income biological fathers' involvement in their toddlers' lives: the Early Head Start National Research and Evaluation Study, *Fathering: A Journal of Theory, Research, and Practice about Men as Fathers*, 2(1), 5–30.

Cabrera, N., Tamis-LeMonda, C., Bradley, R., Hofferth, S. & Lamb, M. (2000) Fatherhood in the 21st century, *Child Development*, 71, 127–136.

Casper, L. M. & O'Connell, M. (1998) Work, income, the economy and married fathers as childcare providers, *Demography*, 35, 243–250.

Coltrane, S. (2004) Fathering: paradoxes, contradictions, and dilemmas, in: M. Coleman & L. Ganong (Eds) *Handbook of contemporary families: considering the past, contemplating the future* (Thousand Oaks, CA, Sage), 224–243.

Cummings, E. M. & O'Reilly, A. W. (1997) Fathers in family context: effects of marital quality on child development, in: M. E. Lamb (Ed.) *The role of the father in child development* (New York, Wiley), 49–65.

Davis, E. C. & Friel, L. V. (2001) Adolescent sexuality: disentangling the effects of family structure and family context, *Journal of Marriage and Family*, 63, 669–681.

Day, R. D. & Lamb, M. E. (2004) Pathways, problems, and progress, in: R. D. Day & M. E. Lamb (Eds) *Conceptualizing and measuring father involvement* (Hillsdale, NJ, Erlbaum), 1–15.

Donate-Bartfield, D. & Passman, R. H. (1985) Attentiveness of mothers and fathers to their baby's cries, *Infant Behavior & Development*, 8, 385–393.

Durkin, D. (1966) *Children who read early* (New York, Teachers College Press).

Ehrenreich, B. & English, D. (1979) *For her own good* (New York, Anchors Books).

Fagan, J. (2000) Head Start fathers' daily hassles and involvement with their children, *Journal of Family Issues*, 21(3), 329–346.

Fagan, J. & Iglesias, A. (1999) Father involvement program effects on fathers, father figures, and their head start children: a quasi-experimental study, *Early Childhood Research Quarterly*, 14(2), 243–269.

Furstenberg, F. F. (1995) Fathering in the inner city: paternal participation and public policy, in: W. Marsiglio (Ed.) *Fatherhood: contemporary theory, research, and social policy* (Thousand Oaks, CA, Sage), 119–147.

Gable, S., Crnic, K. & Belsky, J. (1994) Coparenting with the family system: influences on children's development, *Family Relations*, 43, 380–386.

Gadsden, V. L., Fagan, J., Ray, A. & Davis, J. E. (2004) Fathering indicators for practice and evaluation: the fathering indicators framework, in: R. D. Day & M. E. Lamb (Eds) *Conceptualizing and measuring father involvement* (Hillsdale, NJ, Erlbaum), 385–415.

Gerson, K. (1993) *No man's land: men's changing commitments to family and work* (New York, Basic Books).

Green, S. (2003) Reaching out to fathers: an examination of staff efforts that lead to greater father involvement in early childhood programs, *Early Childhood Research & Practice*, 5(2). Available online at: http://ecrp.uiuc.edu/v5n2/green.html (accessed 1 January 2006).

Hawkins, A. J. & Dollahite, D. C. (1997) *Generative fathering: beyond the deficit perspective* (Thousand Oaks, CA, Sage).

Jaffee, S. R., Moffitt, T. E., Caspi, A. & Taylor, A. (2003) Life with (or without) father: the benefits of living with two biological parents depend on the father's antisocial behavior, *Child Development*, 74(1), 109–126.

Kesner, J. E. & McKenry, P. C. (2001) Single parenthood and social competence in children of color, *Families in Society*, 82(2), 136–143.

Lamb, M. E. (2000) The history of research on father involvement: an overview, in: H. E. Peters, G. W. Peterson, S. K. Steinmetz & R. D. Day (Eds) *Fatherhood: research, interventions and policies* (New York, Haworth Press), 23–44.

Lamb, M. E. (2004) *The role of the father in child development* (New York, Wiley).

Lamb, M. E., Pleck, J. H., Charnov, E. L. & Levine, J. A. (1985) Paternal behavior in humans, *American Zoologist*, 25, 883–894.

LaRossa, R. (1997) *The modernization of fatherhood: a social and political history* (Chicago, IL, University of Chicago Press).

LaRossa, R. & Reitzes, D. C. (1993) Symbolic interactionism and family studies, in: P. G. Boss, W. J. Doherty, R. LaRossa, W. R. Schumm & S. K. Steinmetz (Eds) *Sourcebook of family theories and methods: a contextual approach* (New York, Plenum), 135–163.

Levine, J. A., Murphy, D. T. & Wilson, S. (1993) *Getting men involved* (New York, Scholastic).

Levy-Shiff, R. & Israelashvili, R. (1988) Antecedents of fathering: some further exploration, *Developmental Psychology*, 24, 434–440.

Marks, L. & Palkovitz, R. (2004) American fatherhood types: the good, the bad, and the uninterested, *Fathering*, 2(2), 113–129.

Morman, M. T. & Floyd, K. (2002) A 'changing culture of fatherhood': effects on affectionate communication, closeness, and satisfaction in men's relationships with their fathers and their sons, *Western Journal of Communication*, 66, 395–411.

Nord, C. W., Brimhall, D. & West, J. (1997) *Fathers' involvement in their children's schools* (Washington, DC, U.S. Department of Education). Available online at: http://nces.ed.gov/pubs98/98091.pdf (accessed 12 January 2008).

Ortiz, R. W. (2004) Hispanic/Latino fathers and children literacy development examining involvement practices from a sociocultural context, *Journal of Latinos and Education*, 3(3), 165–180.

Ortiz, R. W. & Ordoñez-Jasis, R. (2005) Leyendo juntos (reading together): new directions for Latino parents' early literacy involvement, *Reading Teacher*, 59(2), 110–121.

Ortiz, R. W., Stile, S. & Brown, C. (1999) Early literacy activities of fathers: reading and writing with young children, *Young Children*, 54, 16–18.

Palkovitz, R. (1997) Reconstructing 'involvement': expanding conceptualizations of men's caring in contemporary families, in: A. J. Hawkins & D. C. Dollahite (Eds) *Generative fathering: beyond a deficit perspective* (Thousand Oaks, CA, Sage), 200–216.

Palkovitz, R. (2002) Involved fathering and child development: advancing our understanding of good fathering, in: C. S. Tamis-LeMonda & N. Cabrera (Eds) *Handbook of father involvement: multidisciplinary perspectives* (Hillsdale, NJ, Erlbaum), 119–140.

Palkovitz, R. & Palm, G. (2005) Transitions within fathering, paper presented at the *Theory Construction and Research Methodology Workshop*, National Council on Family Relations, Phoenix, AZ, 15 November.

Parke, R. D. (1996) *Fatherhood* (Cambridge, MA, Harvard University Press).

Parke, R. D. (2000) Father involvement: a developmental psychological perspective, *Marriage & Family Review*, 29, 43–58.

Parke, R. D. & Buriel, R. (1997) Socialization in the family: ethnic and ecological perspectives, in: N. Eisenberg (Ed.) & W. Damon (Series Ed.) *Handbook of child psychology: social, emotional, and personality development* (vol. 3, 5th edn) (New York, Wiley), 463–552.

Pleck, E. H. & Pleck, J. H. (1997) Fatherhood ideals in the United States: historical dimensions, in: M. E. Lamb (Ed.) *The role of the father in child development* (3rd edn) (New York, Wiley), 33–48.

Pleck, J. H. (1997) Paternal involvement: levels, sources, and consequences, in: M. E. Lamb (Ed.) *The role of the father in child development* (3rd edn) (New York, Wiley), 66–103.

Pleck, J. H. & Masciadrelli, B. P. (2004) Paternal involvement by U.S. residential fathers, in: M. E. Lamb (Ed.) *The role of the father in child development* (4th edn) (New York, Wiley), 222–271.

Presser, H. (1995) Job, family and gender: determinants of non-standard work schedules among employed Americans in 1991, *Demography*, 32, 577–598.

Rohner, R. P. & Veneziano, R. A. (2001) The importance of father love: history and contemporary evidence, *Review of General Psychology*, 5(4), 382–405.

Russell, G. (1983) *The changing roles of fathers* (St. Lucia, Queensland, University of Queensland Press).

Saracho, O. N. (2007a) Hispanic father–child sociocultural literacy practices, *Journal of Hispanic Higher Education*, 6(3), 272–283.

Saracho, O. N. (2007b) Fathers and young children's literacy experiences, *Early Child Development and Care*, 177(4), 403–415.

Schoppe-Sullivan, S. J., McBride, B. A. & Ho, M. R. (2004) Unidimensional versus multidimensional perspectives on father involvement, *Fathering: A Journal of Theory, Research, and Practice about Men as Fathers*, 2, 147–163.

Shannon, J., Tamis-LeMonda, C. S., London, K. & Cabrera, N. (2002) Beyond rough and tumble: low-income fathers' interactions and children's cognitive development at 24 months, *Parenting: Science and Practice*, 2(2), 77–104.

Stile, S. & Ortiz, R. W. (1999) A model for involvement of fathers in literacy development with young at-risk and exceptional children, *Early Childhood Education Journal*, 26(4), 221–224.

Stolz, L. (1954) *Father relations of war-born children* (Stanford, CA, Stanford University Press) (Reprinted, New York, Greenwood Press 1968).

Stryker, S. & Statham, A. (1985) Symbolic interactionism and role theory, in: G. Linzey & E. Aronson (Eds) *Handbook of social psychology* (New York, Random House), 311–378.

Tamis-LeMonda, C. S. & Cabrera, N. J. (2002) Multidisciplinary perspectives on father involvement, in: C. S. Tamis-LeMonda & N. J. Cabrera (Eds) *Handbook of father involvement: multidisciplinary perspectives* (Hillsdale, NJ, Erlbaum), xi–xviii.

Tamis-LeMonda, C. S., Shannon, J. D., Cabrera, N. J. & Lamb, M. E. (2004) Fathers and mothers at play with their 2- and 3-year-olds: contributions to language and cognitive development, *Child Development*, 75(6), 1806–1820.

Taylor, B. A. & Behnke, A. (2005) Fathering across the border: Latino fathers in Mexico and the U.S., *Fathering: A Journal of Theory, Research & Practice about Men as Fathers*, 3(2), 99–120.

Fathers' and young children's literacy experiences

Olivia N. Saracho
University of Maryland, USA

Introduction

Recently, researchers have begun exploring fathers' involvement in early childhood programs (Fagan, 2000; Lamb, 2004), especially in two major research domains: (1) the relationship between child developmental outcomes and patterns of fathers' involvement and absence (e.g., Lamb, 2004); and (2) the ways fathers balance economic provisions, household work, and participation in child-rearing practices (e.g., Palkovitz, 2002; Coltrane, 2004; Marks & Palkovitz, 2004). Limited research on fathers' involvement in their children's lives (Levine, Murphy, & Wilson, 1993) may have resulted in fathers not being perceived as significant contributors to their children's development.

Presently, fathers' involvement with their children is receiving considerable interest. Inquiry in this area may have emerged as a result of the modifications in women's work patterns and men's personal interest in engaging in child care (Gerson, 1993; Parke, 1996). These studies indicated that fathers assume an important role in their children's development. Children whose fathers continuously participated and encouraged them achieved (1) better school performance (Nord *et al.*, 1997), (2) good self-esteem, (3) healthier relationships with peers, (4) healthier sex-role development (Green, 2003), (5) higher academic achievement (Nord *et al.*, 1997), and (6) better personal success. In addition, evidence indicates that fathers' involvement has important implications for several family members. Therefore, fathers need to be perceived as part of a family support system.

Family literacy roles

Researchers, scholars, professional organizations, and educators have underscored the importance of family participation, interest, and support that contribute to the children's school achievement (Barillas, 2000). Family members provide a foundation to develop literacy skills early in their children's lives when they coo, sing lullabies, match letter sounds with letter names, or read to the children (U.S. Department of Education, 2000). Parents are generally attentive to their children's learning from birth (Cairney, 2000). In many cases, family members periodically read to children, model reading to children, make reading and writing materials accessible to children, and stimulate children to raise and respond to questions (Saracho, 2002b).

Regardless of the strong support that families contribute to their children's school performance, only a few studies have been conducted on family literacy and parental support in the children's literacy development. These studies have mostly examined maternal contributions (Ortiz, 2004). They have viewed mothers as primary caregivers and have assumed that teaching young children to read and write was primarily the mothers' responsibility (Dickinson *et al.*, 1992). In addition, studies indicated changes in traditional family structures as an explanation for the problems of home environments. For example, fathers were found to be absent from family life because of changes in family make-up (e.g., higher divorce rates, dramatically increased numbers of out-of-wedlock births, neglect), which challenges the schools (Blankenhorn, 1995). Fathers, who are part of the family, were seen as too busy elsewhere to participate in their children's literacy development. In attempting to determine fathers' role in their young children's reading achievement in elementary school, Durkin (1966) found it impossible to get fathers to show up for interviews to discuss their role in early reading activities. Their excuses consisted of 'being on the road,' 'working during the day and going to school at night,' 'spending long hours at the office,' and 'having two jobs.' Few fathers who were interviewed seemed to have some positive influence on their children's early reading achievement.

The case

The few studies examining the role of fathers in their children's literacy development have suggested that paternal early literacy activities range from fathers who rarely read with their children to those who establish consistent reading and writing routines (Ortiz, 1994, 2004). Marks and Palkovitz (2004) emphasised that families need to have an appropriate balance in involving fathers. They suggested that existing research on the fathers' involvement has been frequently taken for granted, holds negative connotations, and has been inadequately conceptualised.

Fathers can be provided with interesting and motivating opportunities for them to assume responsibility to promote their children's literacy development. The literature indicated that fathers would engage in their children's literacy development when given opportunities to do things that are interesting (Whittenmore, 1992; Ortiz, 1994, 2004; Ortiz *et al.*, 1999; Stile & Ortiz, 1999). Ortiz and his colleagues (e.g., Ortiz *et al.*, 1999; Stile & Ortiz, 1999; Ortiz, 2004) discussed different methods that fathers can use to become involved with their children's literacy. They suggested a variety of reading and writing activities with which the father–child dyads can become involved. They also provided recommendations for teachers who wish to initiate and support literacy activities with fathers and children in their classrooms. Their involvement can influence their children's literacy learning. A literacy program for fathers can help them learn literacy strategies that they can use in a family environment. Thus, they can become critical contributors to their children's literacy development.

Purpose of the study

Since limited research is available on fathers' contributions to their children's reading and writing development, the purpose of this study was to develop and examine the success of an intervention program intended to enhance fathers' support of their children's literacy since such a study has not been conducted before. Since the literature indicated that fathers would engage in their children's literacy development when given opportunities to do things that are interesting, this study identified approaches that could work with fathers which differed from those that have been used with mothers. The identification of strategies that fathers can use can fill in the gap on how fathers can contribute to their children's acquisition of literacy.

This study describes the findings and implications from a case study concerning the literacy experiences in a family environment of 25 fathers who participated in a literacy program. What follows is an attempt to characterise the methodology of case studies in relation to the research process, the formulation of emerging trends and innovations as well as the negotiated understanding of the program that constituted the object of study. Research efforts to understand the fathers' contributions to their children's literacy development as well as intervention efforts that assist fathers to promote their children's literacy learning were examined.

Case study design

A case study is an intensive study of a single unit with a goal to generalise across a larger set of units. Case studies depend on the same type of co-variational evidence that is used in non-case study research. Thus, the case study method is a specific technique that is used to define cases rather than analyse them (Gerring, 2004). In a case study, the methodology draws attention to what specifically can be learned from the single case. This was the methodology used in this study. It represents a method of learning about a complex instance through description and contextual analysis. A case study is an empirical inquiry that investigates a contemporary phenomenon (1) within its real-life context; (2) when the boundaries between the phenomenon and context are not clearly evident; and (3) in which multiple sources of evidence are used (Yin, 2003).

The use of this methodology makes sense when the contextual conditions are an important component of the phenomenon of interest. Stake (2005) viewed the case study approach as providing the researcher with opportunities to study a contemporary phenomenon. He defined a 'case' as a bounded system of behavioral patterns. In a case, a choice of object to be studied is defined by interest in individual cases.

The case itself may be descriptive of what has already taken place or is currently taking place, or it may be an intervention in enacting changes to be studied and documented (Stevenson, 2004). In case study methodology, data are collected using observations, interviews, and documentary analysis to construct a detailed account of a single or multiple cases (Yin, 2003; Stevenson, 2004; Stake, 2005).

In case study methodology, researchers may assume a number of different roles concerning the object of study, in this case, the fathers' literacy program. These roles may have to do with conducting research (interpreter), offering expert advice (consultant), providing training (teacher), collecting biographies (narrator), evaluating the program, and becoming an assessor of merits and values (Stake, 1995).

In this study, the researcher assumed all of these roles as this particular case study required that the data not only be collected but also be interpreted. Advice was offered to the teachers as needed. Training on literacy and working with fathers was also provided to the teachers. The information collected was written in a narrative form. In addition, the worth of the program was assessed. In assuming all of these roles, the researcher depicted a unique picture on the implementation of the literacy program and its innovations. Although the researcher was ultimately responsible for the research work produced, her role as interpreter of the reality was based on the interpretations given by the participants who were the protagonists. The researcher continuously checked with the participants to verify their interpretations. Thus, the researcher described and analyzed the fathers' literacy program and its innovations based on the perceptions of fathers, children, and teachers.

The program

The participants were 25 fathers of five-year-old children in public school kindergarten classrooms, their kindergarten children, and five teachers of these children who lived within a two-mile radius of the elementary school. This school had one of the largest enrollments in the school district. The fathers and teachers volunteered to participate in the literacy program. The fathers agreed to attend a literacy workshop twice a week for a five-month period; while the teachers agreed to participate in a five-month training program prior to the implementation of the fathers' literacy program.

The kindergarten teachers in the study provided 'traditional' literacy materials, strategies, and activities in their classroom that they had designed themselves. They believed that their approach to literacy focused on the children's literacy development. It was the classroom children[1] themselves who, in the interviews, identified this type of classroom as being an instructional factor.

Researcher:	Of all of these activities, which do you think are the ones that help you learn to read?
Joshua:	Well, those in which you have to think the most. They aren't hard activities, but you have to think hard.
Mary:	There are some activities that at the start you don't understand, but later on you know what to do and do your work right.
Mike:	Many of the activities you have to do, we do not know why, and are not fun.
Researcher:	This morning the teacher said that you had to learn some things. What do you think about this work?
Jane:	But it's different. When you learn to read, you need to memorize some things to put letters together.
Nikki:	The teacher gives us activities that we have do. It is part of school.
Matt:	These activities we also have to do at home. They are not fun 'cause they are for learning.

The purpose of the activities can be summed up, as Joshua expressed it, as providing you with help to make you think. These classrooms are the places where changes are brought together: (1) the conceptual change implied by the assumption that children construct their own learning process; and (2) the methodological change that gives priority to their involvement in the shape of a variety of teaching and learning-reading strategies. Matt's comment suggested that the activities that were provided to the children assumed an important role. Therefore, it was important that a literacy program for the fathers would encourage children's thinking to develop their literacy learning as well as be enjoyable. This required an innovative literacy program which, through the use of simple practice group sessions, would promote learning and the comprehension of literacy concepts.

The fathers in this study were provided with a program that focused on skills that would contribute to a better understanding of their children's literacy development. A faculty member from a university reading center conducted a five-month workshop with the teachers during which teachers developed literacy materials, identified literacy strategies, and planned appropriate literacy activities that would help fathers to learn strategies that would promote their children's literacy development. Teachers also learned ways to recruit and retain fathers into the program, establish rapport with them, and motivate their learning.

During the next five months, teachers conducted literacy workshops with fathers, which were held twice a week. Teachers introduced and demonstrated literacy strategies and activities. Fathers learned to cultivate their children's literacy in a family environment by reading culture- and family-related books to their children, engaging their children in discussion about the books they read, recording on a notebook the books they read, and encouraging children to read more books. When fathers and children needed to practice literacy strategies and activities together, children accompanied their fathers to the literacy workshops.

The process

Data collection

In case study methodology, data are collected using observations, interviews, and documentary analysis to construct a detailed account of a single or multiple cases (Yin, 2003; Stevenson, 2004; Stake, 2005). This case study used these procedures to focus on a literacy program that was examined under natural conditions. The teachers provided fathers with a literacy program that they could use in their family environment. The study provided a description of the learning process through observations, samples of children's work, photographs, and in-depth periodic interviews with children, fathers, and teachers. In addition, samples of children's stories were collected, field notes were recorded in a notebook, photographs were taken, and sketches were drawn throughout the study.

The workshops and the fathers' interactions with their children, other fathers, and teachers were videotaped. In addition, fathers selected, presented, and shared literacy strategies and activities with other fathers, teachers, and researchers. Fathers were also interviewed at the beginning and the end of (1) the program, (2) each workshop, and (3) the demonstration activities.

Videotaped observations and interviews were transcribed, typed, and summarised. A summary description was made of each dyad (father and child). Dyad profiles were analysed qualitatively for interaction patterns that might illuminate the cultural contexts in their home, their literacy skills, their knowledge of resources, and their beliefs about literacy.

Father–child interactions in relation to their choice of literacy strategies and activities were the primary units of analysis. The workshops and the reported literacy experiences in the home environment were culled from the profiles, which indicated that the literacy program provided fathers of young children with new skills that contributed to their greater understanding of literacy development. The program components integrated both the home and school conventional and non-conventional strategies for literacy development.

The data provided a unique picture of the implementation of the fathers' literacy program as well as of innovations and trends in particular contexts. These data were bound to their specific contexts and could be used in answering the program's general questions. In this way, an argument was formulated based on those aspects of the case that lent themselves to describing and analysing the fathers' literacy program according to the perceptions of fathers, children, and teachers.

Verification

Operational definitions provided verification, narratives, or representations of the concepts that had been extracted from separate conceivable phenomena based on the focus of the study. These operational definitions were used to assess the accuracy of the verification, narratives, or representations of the concepts. The operational definitions were identified from the literature on emergent literacy. Since it was essential that the same definitions were in the participants' minds, during the workshops, operational definitions were stated and explained in a way that both the researcher and participants understood the meaning.

It was imperative that the inferences be tested with participants. Fathers were interviewed before and at the end of each workshop and/or during demonstration to verify the observer's inferences. The observer shared these inferences with the participants. Inferences that were considered valid were those that were confirmed (1) by the participants, and (2) by cross-referencing different sets of data. In addition, fathers had a comprehensive exit interview at the completion of the literacy program. They examined the data and explained any misconceptions that were constructed during the data collection. They also accounted for their choices of specific behaviors and answered the researcher's questions.

Identifying innovations and trends

Descriptive inference remains an important, often undervalued, rhetorical device within the social sciences. A methodological affinity exists between descriptive inference and case study work. When describing a phenomenon one is usually comparing it to an ideal-type that conforms to standard perceptions. Typically, a genre of descriptive case study maintains that the unit under study is like, or unlike, other similar units (Gerring, 2004; Stake, 2005).

One of the most interesting factors in this case study was each of the participants' unique approach to their children's literacy development. Each resorted to different styles of using home materials and experiences, even in their initial stages. The following quotations show each case in relation to an innovation (or a series of innovations) generally incorporated in the teaching/learning strategies that were taught to the fathers in the literacy program.

These quotations show the specific innovations and may be of help in understanding such innovations. The fathers described the learning process as follows:

Tim: We talk about real problems and we try to use literacy to teach reading and make our problems easy. Like we talk about the activities we learned at the workshop and how we use them at home. One of us will tell other fathers what we did and that father sometimes thinks of a way he can use the same activity for a different reason. Like in the workshop we learned to use foil paper to make a moon and stars for the story *Papa, Please Get the Moon for Me*. Since we do not use foil paper at home, I used plain white paper because the moon and stars are white.

Manny: I am going to try it, because we do not have foil paper either. We also do not have binoculars to look at the moon. I used two construction papers, rolled

> them so that we can see through them, glued them, and then looked at the
> moon at night.
>
> Fred: Can we get together on Sunday afternoon, watch the game, and then share
> what we have done with the activities at home?

The quotations above suggest innovations and trends related to the learning in the literacy program:

- *Teaching-learning process*: Fathers shared how they were using what they had learned by teaching other fathers different ways of using the strategies and activities they learned in the literacy program.
- *Collaboration*: Fathers organised and worked in a collaborative way in the literacy program.

It can be inferred that fathers could make important contributions if they learned literacy strategies and activities that would promote their children's literacy development in a family environment. To provide a clear description of the literacy program and a view from the participants' frame of reference, many quotations and examples from the participants are provided in a narrative form. These are presented in the succeeding sections.

Strategies and activities

Fathers practiced at home the strategies and activities that they learned in the workshop. In addition, they extended these literacy strategies and activities to match their interests, concerns, and environment in both the family and community settings. This outcome was observed in the fathers' literacy demonstrations where they shared strategies and activities that they felt comfortable with.

In examining the data on the literacy workshops, presentations, activities, and writing experiences, fathers usually used materials that were found in both the family and community settings including:

- *Non-print materials* that had a visual incentive (e.g., spider puppet, cowboy hat, comic strips, photographs) to expand and compose a story.
- *Print materials* (e.g., children's books, newspapers, magazines) that had a visual incentive to motivate them to create stories.
- *Library materials* that included children's books from the school and public library as well as pictures (photographs or magazine pictures) that were relevant to the family, community, and school situations.
- *No materials* were used. Fathers depended on conversations that would motivate oral and written language. Interactions with others provided the fathers and children opportunities (e.g., sharing an interesting story with others) to interact with adults or other children to promote their vocabulary and knowledge.

The materials fathers used were (1) children's books related to their concerns and interests (such as family photographs or comic strips), (2) magazine pictures that could be used in writing stories, and (3) objects found in the family and community environment that related to the children's books that were used for an activity. The use of these materials reflected the resourcefulness of the fathers in using a variety of materials from different resources to become involved in their children's early literacy development.

Literacy workshops

The teachers developed lesson plans for each workshop to help fathers promote literacy learning. A university faculty member was a consultant and periodically met with the teacher who served as the coordinator of the workshop. The teachers in these workshops focused on using materials found in home and community, such as popsicle sticks, paper grocery bags, fruits, vegetables, and photographs. Neither the teachers nor the fathers were required to buy any special materials. Teachers taught fathers how to select books, tell a story, and engage children in related activities that would promote their children's literacy development. The purpose of the activities was to guide fathers in teaching children to construct their own learning process and develop a variety of teaching and learning-reading strategies.

Teachers greeted the fathers at the door at the beginning of each workshop session and recorded the names of the fathers who were in attendance. They then invited the fathers and their children (when they were in attendance) to have a snack. These snacks were made available during the entire time of the workshop. They then gathered the fathers together to initiate a literacy activity. The teachers stated the purpose (e.g., monitoring comprehension, language development) of the activity in relation to the children's literacy development. Then they provided the fathers with specific strategies to achieve that purpose. For example, teachers taught the fathers how to (1) select and read a book to their children; (2) engage them in a discussion; (3) use prediction to monitor their understanding of the story or text; and (4) motivate them to write, create, and read their own stories. The teachers would reinforce their instruction by working with the fathers on activities similar to the ones they might use with their children.

In the next workshop session, the fathers would bring their children and engage them in the activities and strategies they had learned in the previous workshop. Teachers also encouraged fathers to create and use different activities that would be of interest to both the fathers and their children and would achieve the same purpose.

At the end of each session, fathers and teachers evaluated the experiences and planned their next session. Fathers were encouraged to bring materials that were of interest to them. For example, a father who worked in a port city brought seashells and sand. They also discussed other strategies they might use and planned for the next workshop session. Fathers typically left in an excited manner, interacting with each other, and discussing their plans to promote their children's literacy development. They talked about books, strategies, and activities they planned to use in their home environment.

Literacy demonstrations

Fathers would engage their children in literacy activities, such as listening to a story, discussing it, developing a related activity, and writing about it. Fathers selected and presented literacy activities that they implemented with their children in a family environment. They demonstrated the use of children's books, literacy strategies, activities, and materials. Most of them shared a children's book, had a conversation about the story, clarified misconceptions, worked on an activity with their child to develop a story, and wrote a related story. For example, *The Fish Who Could Wish* by Bush and Paul (1993) was a book that stimulated Zeke and his father to compose and illustrate a story. This book is about a fish with magical powers. When he makes a wish, it always comes true. The fish makes many wishes such as wishing for a car, new suits with silk ties, a castle, a shark, and, finally, wishing for a plain fish. Zeke and his father worked on an activity. They took large pieces of paper, drew a fish, decorated it, cut two identical size fish, stapled both fish around the edges, stuffed it with newspapers, attached it to a string, and hung it to be mobile. Then they wrote and illustrated the following story.

> *Zeke's story*
> One day he wished for a castle.
> The other day he wished for a car.
> And the other day he went to his grandma to visit her.
> And his dad came early he cried because he wanted to stay but he had school.
> After school he went again to his grandma and his grandma gave him cookies.
> He ate them all and he spended the night at his grandma's house.
> The End

Fathers selected books that were of interest to them (father and child). In addition, they chose books on father and child relationships such as *Papa, Please Get the Moon for Me* by Eric Carle (1991), *Fishing with Dad: Lessons of Love and Lure from Father to Son* by Michael J. Rosen (1996), *When Daddy Came to School* by Julie Brillhart (1995), *What Daddies Do Best* by Laura Nmeroff (1998), and *When Daddy Took Us Camping* by Julie Brillhart (1997).

Writing experiences

In addition to writing stories that related to the books they read, fathers engaged in other writing experiences with children. Children usually dictated stories about their books, family, experiences they had with their fathers, and family photographs. Although fathers recorded the children's dictated stories, they encouraged them to experiment with writing using invented symbols or messages on their illustrations. They wrote about their family experiences including easy family recipes, family events, and family life. The following subsections describe several of their writing experiences.

Family recipes.   Fathers and their children wrote and implemented easy recipes in a family event or a snack. For example, Ralph and his son made peanut butter to spread on their bread for a snack. They used magic markers to write and illustrate the materials and directions for the recipe. Using picture reading, they recorded the following:

How to make peanut butter

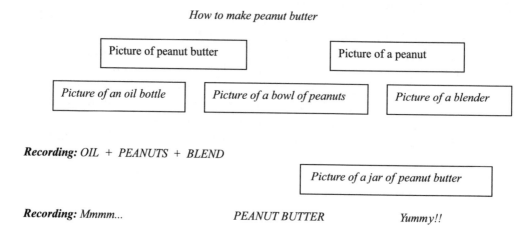

Recording: *OIL + PEANUTS + BLEND*

Recording: *Mmmm...*   *PEANUT BUTTER*   *Yummy!!*

Family events. Fathers engaged in reading and writing activities that provided knowledge in an area of their choice. This knowledge also included the family's culture that, by its disposition, is integrated into fathers' and their children's life situations. Fathers and their children also wrote stories about recent family events. Recently, Amanda had a birthday party. She discussed and dictated this episode to her father:

My birthday
When it's my birthday or anyone's birthday, we usually have a cake and ice cream. I get a piñata like Pocahontas and my brother gets other things.
When we go to the park my father, mom, brother, my aunt and me play in the monkey bars. My brother Hector and me play always. My father, mom and my aunt Theresa eat a snow cone while we play.
We also go to the movies with my dad, aunt Theresa, mom, Hector, my brother, me. After the movies we go home and order pizza to eat at home.
We go visit my grandparents at Dallas and my uncle Bet usually takes us to the park and barbecues fish. He likes cooking.

Family life. Another writing experience was getting the fathers and their children to write and illustrate stories about their family life. For example, the Travis family had gone to Chicago to visit a family member. Karen and her father took to a workshop session some photographs that they had taken on their trip, discussed them, and arranged them in order to create a story. Then Karen dictated the following story to her father:

The Travis family
Once upon a time the Travis Family went to Chicago and we went to each hotel. And we ate breakfast at the hotel. At the hotel we went way up high on the 33rd floor. We were at

Chicago visiting Uncle Leonard and his girlfriend Carrol. And one night we saw Carrol and I said I love you and she cried. And then we went to the hotel and went to bed. The next day we went to the Cirque Du Soliel. We all had a good time and I was always happy when we went back to the hotel. And then we ate lunch and we went on a big boat touring Chicago. Then my brother and me got cookies and drinks on the boat. Then we went to eat at Fat Tuesdays and me and my brother got a cherry drink, kind of like an Icee. And my brother bought Yacko. The next day we went to a museum. Then we came home.

The writing experiences exposed young children to patterns of reading and writing. It seemed that the children engaged in written language activities. When fathers and children composed many different texts, they experienced many types of writing systems. These writing behaviors may have helped young children to become aware of the relationship between language and print.

Program perceptions

At the end of the literacy program, fathers had exit interviews with the researcher. The results indicated two major differences: (1) different fathers favored different literacy strategies, and (2) fathers differed in their perceptions of the benefit of the literacy program. Each father seemed to have benefitted from the literacy intervention program and each of them expressed a positive response. For example, the following are some of the fathers' reactions to the literacy intervention program:

Mr. Z.:   I liked it a lot, because I saw that many fathers are interested in their children and the children want to learn a lot.

Mr. M.:   For me, it has been a beautiful experience with my daughter, because she is the only one I have and I have gained something. Thank you, because it is her first here and I am very proud of her.

Mr. C.:   For me, it has been a beautiful experience. I have been with my daughter telling stories. I think she progressed in reading a lot.

Mr. G.:   In my house, my boy, Isaac has older brothers and all since they were little were used to reading.

Fathers seemed very positive about the literacy program. Its approaches were innovative for the fathers. Literacy workshops and demonstrations also provided similar evidence. They also suggested a heuristic framework within which the home environment can be analysed and discussed, and could augment the meaning of family socialisation and family strengths. The fathers' quotations showed each case in relation to the teaching/learning strategies that the fathers learned in the literacy program. Their quotations suggested trends and innovations related to their learning in the literacy program.

The above trends and innovations indicated that fathers could make important contributions if they learned literacy strategies and activities that would promote their children's literacy development in a family environment. To provide a clear description of the literacy program and a view from the participants' frame of reference, several quotations and examples from the participants were provided in a narrative form. These were presented in the preceding sections.

Challenges and limitations

All approaches to research have challenges and limitations. It is important to share those that were confronted in this study, especially in relation to collaboration, recruiting, and retaining participants. The main challenge dealt with the need to have all participants collaborate. Collaboration is essential in case study research (Christie *et al.*, 2004). Retention of participants is a critical element for success in a collaborative case study. Collaboration relies on, and is defined by, the constant negotiation of roles, meanings, and goals. Pivotal to this process is the continuous interaction of the participants (Gerring, 2004; Stake, 2005). Although all the participants remained in the study until the completion of the program, it was a constant struggle to keep them interested enough to continue. The success may be attributed, at least in part, to the consistent enthusiasm of the teachers who generated activities that would be of interest to the fathers. For example, activities that focused on sports were used to sustain the interest of those fathers who were interested in sports. The sessions were planned and evaluated with the fathers to identify future topics that were of interest to them. The scheduling (date and time) of the workshop and demonstrations were also planned with them to avoid conflict of family responsibilities or events. Also snacks were provided for those fathers who had rushed from work and had not had time to enjoy their dinner at their leisure. Fathers also enjoyed the many opportunities they had to interact with each other to exchange literacy ideas and share family problems.

Another important limitation is that the observations and other collections of the data were conducted from the 'inside' (Christie *et al.*, 2004). That is, the researcher developed the literacy program as well as recorded the notes, exchanges, and observations to document this process instead of having an outside observer. The subjective nature of this kind of work needs to be acknowledged. On the other hand, continuous verification and triangulation were used to ensure that the descriptive inferences were grounded in data rather than speculation. Inferences were continuously checked. For example, patterns and categories that were identified in the data would be verified with at least two other types of evidence, hypotheses, and member checks. In addition, rival explanations to the data were considered and then those who were involved directly and indirectly responded to the data and the analysis. Finally, a draft of this report was shared with the participants for any reactions and comments.

The collaborative process, described above, seemed to be important to share. Collaboration throughout the case study seemed to have had positively impacted the productivity of the literacy program and participants.

Conclusion

Outcomes from both the literacy workshops and fathers' literacy demonstrations indicated which strategies fathers used with the literacy-related activities. The clusters delineated above characterised the literacy activities that fathers and children implemented in a family environment. They also suggested a heuristic framework within which the home environment can be analysed and discussed, and could augment the meaning of family socialisation and family strengths.

Fathers, like mothers, can be responsible for the development of their children's literacy and writing skills. They can serve as resources and meaning-makers in their children's family environment. Marks and Palkovitz (2004) suggested that the fathers' roles be conceptualised to help families have an appropriate balance in their involvement. Ortiz (2004) provided evidence of paternal involvement and the themes that tend to drive these practices. Ortiz and his colleagues (e.g., Ortiz *et al.*, 1999; Stile & Ortiz, 1999) recommended a variety of reading and writing activities to promote father–child dyads. Several of their suggestions were implemented in this study.

Teachers must be aware of the community and families' beliefs, attitudes, and roles in their children's literacy development when they work closely with families. According to Nistler and Maiers (2000), Saracho (2002a), and Tett (2000), teachers need to use literacy practices in relation to what families already know and do in their home and community. They have found that families browsed the television guides' program daily schedule, read their horoscopes, read signs and symbols in their local environment, wrote brief notes to other family members, developed shopping lists, labeled family photographs, identified family birthdays and anniversaries, wrote greeting cards, and conversed with others. Many times, family members occasionally read to children, modeled reading to children, made reading and writing materials accessible to children, and motivated children to raise and respond to questions (Saracho, 2002a).

Studies have noted that young children learn to read when families provided literacy-rich environments, experiences, and interactions. Families need to provide children with the opportunity to access books that will enhance their perception of competence with print (Barnes *et al.*, 2000). These studies suggest that fathers were able to motivate children to acquire, develop, and use literacy and also supported the idea that fathers can learn new roles to promote their children's literacy development.

Note

1. Pseudonyms have been substituted for the names of participants to protect their privacy.

References

Barillas, M. D. R. (2000) Literacy at home: honoring parent voices through writing, *Reading Teacher*, 53(3), 302–308.

Barnes, W. S., Snow, C. E., Hemphill, L., Chandler, J. & Goodman, I. F. (2000) *Unfulfilled expectations: home and school influences on literacy* (Cambridge, Harvard University Press).

Blankenhorn, D. (1995) *Fathers in America* (New York, Basic Books).

Cairney, T. H. (2000) Beyond the classroom walls: the rediscovery of the family and community as partners in education, *Educational Review*, 52(2), 163–172.

Christie, C. A., Ross, R. M. & Klein, B. M. (2004) Moving toward collaboration by creating a participatory internal–external evaluation team: a case study, *Studies in Educational Evaluation*, 30, 125–134.

Coltrane, S. (2004) Fathering: paradoxes, contradictions, and dilemmas, in: M. Coleman & L. Ganong (Eds) *Handbook of contemporary families: considering the past, contemplating the future* (Thousand Oaks, CA, Sage), 224–243.

Dickinson, D. K., De Temple, J. M. & Smith, M. W. (1992) Book reading with preschoolers: construction of text at home and at school, *Early Childhood Research Quarterly*, 7, 323–346.

Durkin, D. (1966) *Children who read early* (New York, Teachers College Press).

Fagan, J. (2000) Head Start fathers' daily hassles and involvement with their children, *Journal of Family Issues*, 21(3), 329–346.

Gerring, J. (2004) What is a case study and what is it good for? *American Political Science Review*, 98(2), 341–354.

Gerson, K. (1993) *No man's land: men's changing commitments to family and work* (New York, Basic Books).

Green, S. (2003) Reaching out to fathers: an examination of staff efforts that lead to greater father involvement in early childhood programs, *Early Childhood Research and Practice*, 5(2). Available online at: http://ecrp.uiuc.edu/v5n2/green.html (accessed 1 January 2006).

Lamb, M. E. (2004) *The role of the father in child development* (New York, John Wiley).

Levine, J. A., Murphy, D.T. & Wilson, S. (1993) *Getting men involved* (New York, Scholastic).

Marks, L. & Palkovitz, M. R. (2004) American fatherhood types: the good, the bad, and the uninterested, *Fathering*, 2(2), 113–129.

Nistler, R. J. & Maiers, A. (2000) Stopping the silence: hearing parents' voices in an urban first-grade family literacy program, *Reading Teacher*, 53(8), 670–680.

Nord, C. W., Brimhall, D. & West, J. (1997) *Fathers' involvement in their children's schools* (Washington, DC, U.S. Department of Education).

Ortiz, R. W. (1994) Fathers and children explore literacy, *Kamehameha Journal of Education*, 5, 131–134.

Ortiz, R. W. (2004) Hispanic/Latino fathers and children literacy development examining involvement practices from a sociocultural context, *Journal of Latinos and Education*, 3(3), 165–180.

Ortiz, R. W., Stile, S. & Brown, C. (1999) Early literacy activities of fathers reading and writing and young children, *Young Children*, 54(5), 16–18.

Palkovitz, R. (2002) Involved fathering and child development: advancing our understanding of good fathering, in: C. S. Tamis-LeMonda & N. Cabrera (Eds) *Handbook of father involvement: multidisciplinary perspectives* (Hillsdale, NJ, Lawrence Erlbaum), 119–140.

Parke, R. D. (1996) *Fatherhood* (Cambridge, MA, Harvard University Press).

Saracho, O. N. (2002a) Family literacy: exploring family practices, *Early Child Development and Care*, 172(2), 113–122.

Saracho, O. N. (2002b) Promising perspectives and practices in family literacy, in: O. N. Saracho & B. Spodek (Eds) *Contemporary perspectives in literacy in early childhood education* (vol. 2) (Greenwich, CT, Information Age), 151–169.

Stake, R. E. (1995) *The art of case study research* (Thousand Oaks, CA, Sage).

Stake, R. E. (2005) Qualitative case studies, in: N. K. Denzin & Y. S. Lincoln (Eds) *Handbook of qualitative research* (Thousand Oaks, CA, Sage), 443–466.

Stevenson, R. B. (2004) Constructing knowledge of educational practices from case studies, *Environmental Education Research*, 10(1), 39–51.

Stile, S. & Ortiz, R.W. (1999) A model for involvement of fathers in literacy development with young at-risk and exceptional children, *Early Childhood Education Journal*, 26(4), 221–224.

Tett, L. (2000) Excluded voices: class, culture, and family literacy in Scotland, *Journal of Adolescent and Adult Literacy*, 44(2), 122–128.

U.S. Department of Education (2000) Building literacy skills through early care and education, *Reading in the Early Years: Infancy through Kindergarten*, 7(2), 7–8.

Whittenmore, H. (1992, 27 September) Dads who shaped up a school, *Parade Magazine*, pp. 20–22.

Yin, R. K. (2003) *Case study research: design and methods* (Thousand Oaks, CA, Sage).

Children's literature books

Brillhart, J. (1995) *When daddy came to school* (Morton Grove, IL, Albert Whitman).

Brillhart, J. (1997) *When daddy took us camping* (Morton Grove, IL, Albert Whitman).

Bush, J. & Paul, K. (1993) *The fish who could wish* (Brooklyn, NY, Kane/Miller Book).

Carle, E. (1991) *Papa, please get the moon for me* (New York, Simon & Schuster Children's Publishing).

Numeroff, L. with Munsinger, L. (Illustrator) (1998) *What daddies do best* (New York, Simon & Schuster Children's Publishing).

Rosen, M. J. with Shively, W. (Photographer) (1996) *Fishing with dad: lessons of love and lure from father to son* (New York, Artisan).

Men and motors? Fathers' involvement in children's travel

John Barker
Brunel University, UK

Introduction

Whilst social scientists have explored the increasing number of settings in which young children spend their time (Mayall, 1994; Holloway, 1998), a small but growing body of literature has begun to consider how children travel between these different spaces of childhood. Although the term mobility has been used in a number of ways (e.g. social mobility referring to movement relating to social class), this paper focuses upon spatial mobility, which can be defined as 'the short term, repetitive, movement flows of people, designated as circulation' (Law, 1999, p. 568). Although mobility has been an often undervalued concept in the social sciences, it has become an increasingly central feature of most Western, industrialised societies, since human beings are not rooted entirely in one space or place (Urry, 2000; Beckmann, 2001). Mobility is not generally undertaken for its own sake (although walking or driving for leisure are examples of this), but rather enables accessibility to services, people and culture. Whilst these trends are most immediately identifiable in the developed world, there are more global aspirations for increased travel and communication (Urry, 2000).

As part of the 'new mobilities paradigm', there has been a growing interest in children and mobility. Whilst a body of psychology-based literature addresses the psychological and physiological aspects of how young children learn to walk (see McAllister & Grey, 2006), the growing interest in children's mobility is often more externally focused upon children's travel outside of the home and the broader social context of travel. Existing research identifies a number of key and inter-related trends in children's mobility in the UK. Firstly, over the past 30 years, children's independent mobility has declined. The proportion of children under the age of 10/11 undertaking specific tasks outside the home (such as crossing main roads or cycling) alone has declined significantly (see Hillman *et al.*, 1990; Valentine & McKendrick, 1997; O'Brien *et al.*, 2000). Secondly, the decline in children's independent spatial mobility corresponds with an increase in the proportion of journeys for which children are escorted by parents. The proportion of primary school children travelling to school unescorted had dropped from 15% in 1989 to 6% in 2005 (DfT, 2005). Parents often escort their children up to a later age, with the transition to secondary school increasingly seen as a watershed in children's independent spatial mobility (Jones & Bradshaw, 2000; O'Brien *et al.*, 2000).

A third related trend in children's mobility is the increasing use of cars to escort children. There has been a decline in the proportion of primary school children walking to school, from 61% in 1988 to 51% in 2006, and a corresponding increase in the proportion driven to school, from 27% in 1988 to 41% in 2006 (DfT, 2007). Despite increasingly high levels of bicycle ownership, few primary school children cycle to school (Hillman *et al.*, 1990; DfT, 2005). Whilst much research focuses on travel to school, less is known about children's travel patterns outside of school, although research suggests that non-school travel is also becoming increasing car-based (Joshi *et al.*, 1999). Jones and Bradshaw (2000) suggest that 64% of primary school children's non-school journeys are undertaken by car, a much higher proportion than for school journeys.

However, there is growing unease regarding children's increasing dependence on cars and a lack of independent mobility (Royal Commission on Environmental Pollution [RCEP], 1994; Meaton & Kingham, 1998; Jones & Bradshaw, 2000). In addition to concerns regarding children's physical health, there are also concerns about the increasing accident rates of 11/12-year olds, who, when beginning to travel to secondary school unaccompanied, are often not used to walking without escort (DfT, 2004). Escorting children to school by car contributes to congestion. At the height of the morning peak hour, up to 18% of cars on urban roads are escorting children to school (Jones & Bradshaw, 2000; DfT, 2004). In response to these issues, a

2010 target has been set for each school to have its own 'School Travel Plan', which typically focuses upon a combination of street engineering, education and training, and initiatives such as the 'Walking Bus', to reduce dependence on cars for the journey to school (Rye, 2002; Barker, 2003).

There is an established body of research which has identified that escorting children to and from school and other places is largely the responsibility of women, as part of the broader range of 'carescapes', that is the wide variety of caring tasks undertaken both within and outside of the domestic sphere (Bowlby et al., 1997; Law, 1999; Dowling, 2000). Despite the increasing proportion of mothers returning to paid employment, women still remain responsible for most caring tasks, including escorting children (Turner & Grieco, 1998; Dowling, 2000; Skinner, 2003; McDowell, 2004).

Whilst research has begun to map how shifting gender relations may impact upon fathers' roles in different aspects of family life, for example, involvement in domestic tasks (Windebank, 2001) or children's education (West et al., 1998), existing literature has neither considered fathers' involvement in children's mobility nor fathers' own accounts of their role (or lack of) in escorting children. As part of mapping fathers' involvement or absence in children's lives (Saracho, 2007) and a growing recognition that fatherhood is being constantly reshaped and renegotiated (Brandth & Kvande, 1998; Mac an Ghaill & Haywood, 2007), it is timely to explore how the changing domestic roles of fathers may create new freedoms and possibilities for fathers to engage in escorting children. It is this gap in research which this paper hopes to contribute to filling.

Methods

The research was conducted in primary schools in five locations in the UK. Three within Buckinghamshire, a predominantly affluent and rural county north west of London, and two within the London Borough of Enfield, a mixed, mostly suburban area on the northern fringe of London. The two authorities have different levels of car ownership—Buckinghamshire has one of the highest levels of car ownership in the UK, whereas Enfield, as a part of Greater London, has levels similar to the national average (DfT, 2004). Each school was at a different stage of developing its own School Travel Plan.

In each of the five schools, questionnaire surveys were distributed to all families. The survey gathered information regarding how children currently travel to school and other places, and how families would like their children to travel. Questions were also asked about who made decisions about how children travel and who escorted children, as well as broader socio-demographic information. A total of 1956 questionnaire surveys were distributed, 1006 of which were returned completed, giving a response rate of 51%.

Twenty-three families took part in the qualitative stage of the research. This involved conducting in-depth interviews with parents and children regarding children's travel, as well as giving children disposable cameras to take pictures of their journeys and diaries to record their movements over a week (see Barker & Weller, 2003 for more discussion). Most research on parenting (e.g. see Windebank, 2001) involves talking to mothers and often does not include fathers' accounts. Although this research aimed to recruit mothers, fathers and children to participate in the study, fathers were very reluctant to take part. Fathers would often say 'you need to talk to my wife, she knows about that kind of thing'. This reluctance of men to participate has also been found by other researchers studying domestic or intimate aspects of men's lives (Butera, 2006), since some men may be uncomfortable discussing such personal topics as this counters popular and hegemonic ideas about masculinities and men's behaviours. Ten per cent ($n = 98$) of the returned surveys were completed by fathers, and only four fathers (out of 23 families) participated in an in-depth interview. This data is complemented by 21 in-depth interviews with mothers, and interviews with 28 children. Therefore, this paper is as much about mothers and children talking about fathers' involvement (or lack of) in children's travel as much as it is about fathers' own experiences of involvement in escorting children.

Distant dads: gender and escorting tasks

Feminist social scientists have long observed that women have the primary responsibility for organising and undertaking care for children (Mayall, 1994; Laurie *et al.*, 1999; McKie *et al.*, 2002). Table 1 identifies which family members had responsibility for making decisions regarding children's travel. It illustrates that in just under half of two-parent families (46%), mothers had the sole responsibility for making children's travel decisions. This was also reflected in the qualitative stage of the research—in five out of 23 families, mothers were entirely responsible for organising children's travel:

> On the whole, it's me, dashing in and out, sorting it out. (Charlie and Pete's Mum, Bucks)

> In the week the vast majority is her (mother). (Daniel's Dad, Bucks)

> Yes ... definitely (me) ... And if it isn't (me) it's because I have set it up, if I'm doing another run (escort trip) or doing something, then I will have set something else up. (Helen's Mum, Enfield)

This was also reflected in other research highlighting that mothers are often responsible for organising and undertaking escort trips as part of the broader range of

Table 1. Parents' involvement in making decisions regarding children's travel

Decisions made by	One-parent families (%)	Two-parent families (%)
Mother only	86 ($n = 85$)	46 ($n = 401$)
Both parents[a]	11 ($n = 10$)	52 ($n = 453$)
Father only	2 ($n = 2$)	1 ($n = 9$)

[a]In the case of lone-parent families, this refers to lone parent and, where relevant, ex-partner.
Note: Chi-squared (χ^2) = 56.656, df = 2, $p = 0.00$.

'carescapes' (Bowlby *et al.*, 1997; Law, 1999; Dowling, 2000). In many of these families, at least in relation to children's travel, fathers were invisible and only mentioned
briefly or seen to have a very indirect influence on children's travel. In one hour-long
interview, one mother made reference to her husband only once and very indirectly.
He was mentioned because his own travel behaviour (using the family car) was seen
to have consequences on children's travel:

> My problem was that my husband goes away, and often takes the car. So we need one.
> (Elizabeth's Mum, Enfield)

As well as illustrating the invisibility of fathers in some families in relation to escorting
children, this also indicates gendered assumptions regarding car use and priorities
(Maxwell, 2001). Cars are seen as more essential for fathers to get to work than
mothers or children to get to school.

However, a complete lack of involvement of fathers was only found in a limited
number of families. Table 1 suggests at least some involvement of fathers in organising and escorting children in just over half (52%) of two-parent families. Furthermore, in 18 of the 23 families taking part in the qualitative stage of the research,
fathers had at least some involvement. This perhaps reflects a shift in gendered carescapes as new roles are being created for fathers within children's lives (Saracho,
2007), mirroring a broader shift in expectations regarding fatherhood from one based
upon absence to one of closeness, proximity to and engagement with children
(Brandth & Kvande, 1998; Castelain-Meunier, 2002).

However, in most of these cases, despite fathers' contributions, they often did not
have overall responsibility for organising or undertaking the escort of children:

> She (makes the decisions). I make suggestions sometimes but mainly it's my wife. (Lucy's
> Dad, Enfield)

Out of the 23 families taking part in the qualitative, in-depth stage of the research, in
only two families fathers had the main responsibility for planning and undertaking the
escort of children. Even in families where fathers participated in decision-making,
women had most responsibility and undertook most escorting. Fathers' involvement
was limited, and in nine out of 23 families, fathers often helped out mostly at weekends:

> Yes. It is usually (me) … my husband is around at the weekend, but it is me who drives
> them around most of the week. He does his bit on Saturday morning when we have to be
> in three directions at once, but it's generally me. (John's Mum, Bucks)

> Yeah, (it's) usually Mum, but at weekends, my Dad. And he takes us to brownies. (Rachel,
> 7, Bucks)

At weekends, families juggled a complex number of domestic tasks. There are three
particular points of interest about fathers' weekend participation in escorting children.
Firstly, although fathers helped out in weekend carescapes, fathers often participated
in specific tasks reflecting a stereotypical gendered division of labour:

> Alan will help, but generally I do it. It just works out that way. He's mowing the lawn or
> doing something else. (Rebecca and David's Mum, Enfield)

Secondly, that most families spoke of fathers 'helping out' by implication reinforces that mothers still have the overall responsibility to organise children's travel and to escort children—a finding also of research exploring other aspects of household tasks (Windebank, 2001; Edwards, 2006). Featherstone (2004) discusses fathers' involvement in terms of engagement, accessibility and responsibility as factors to gauge the level and extent of participation. It is clear that these examples demonstrate engagement, but rarely this extends to responsibility. Whilst many families may aspire to sharing domestic tasks, few actually manage this in practice. To talk of a gender-equal division of tasks is what Castelain-Meunier (2002, p. 192) calls 'egalitarian fraud'.

Thirdly, fathers' participation in escorting children at the weekend was often limited to and centred around special events such as organising trips and driving during family outings, such as holidays, long journeys, or visits to adult friends and relatives. Almost without exception, these special journeys were car-based:

> If we go with Dad, then it's probably because we go to places that are very far away, or if we go on a very long walk. You enjoy going with someone else ... If we go on long journeys, it's always Daddy. (Rachel, 7, Bucks)

> But sometimes if we are going somewhere (special), Daddy sometimes drives. If we go on holiday, Mummy and Daddy take turns, but usually Daddy does it. He drives around a lot. (Sarah, 9, Bucks)

These 'special' trips were often seen as more complex or requiring more driving skills than everyday, routine journeys:

> When we go on holiday, (or) go up to London, he drives then. He drives around much more, he's more confident than I am. (Lydia and Katey's Mum, Bucks)

Miller (2001) discusses how cars are gendered artefacts. Despite some current trends (such as the increasing proportion of women gaining driving licences and owning cars), cars remain embedded within gendered social relations. The accounts here are particularly gendered and place fathers as competent and skilled to organise and lead special trips. This is firstly because, compared to women, there is a greater association between men, masculinities, cars and driving, and cars play a more prominent role in the production of everyday masculinities (Miller, 2001). Secondly, there are powerful gendered assumptions regarding competency for 'special trips' which are seen as technologically complex (Garvey, 2001) and demand greater driving skills. Furthermore, that fathers have the responsibility for special outings reinforces that mothers are responsible for the more mundane, regular and routine journeys which Dowling (2000, p. 347) describes as the 'temporal treadmill', which by implication are seen to require lower skills. Like many other gendered social practices, similar everyday behaviours are refracted as either 'mundane, everyday and unskilled' or 'specialist, complex and demanding' depending at least in part upon the gender of the participant.

Parents offered two main reasons for fathers' limited involvement in escorting children. The primary reason was fathers' involvement in paid employment:

> I don't take them much. I have to leave early in the morning and come back late at night.
> I work on Saturdays too. (Daniel's Dad, Bucks)

> Daddy's at work so doesn't do (the escorting). He's never here during the week, he gets in
> too late. (Rebecca and David's Mum, Enfield)

To return to Featherstone's (2004) discussion, inaccessibility is a crucial factor as fathers are often unable to take part in escorting children due to paid employment. As another example of gendered carescapes, whilst employment was seen as a valid reason to limit the involvement of fathers, women's participation in similar tasks, including full-time employment, rarely released them from their domestic responsibilities (Bowlby et al., 1997). Furthermore, in addition to their absence due to paid employment, fathers were also released from such tasks at other times whilst at home. Fathers were allowed to be 'tired of driving' or 'tired from work' in a way that women were not, suggesting fathers may be able to pursue their own interests above those of the household (Pilcher, 2000). This questions the extent to which broader changes in women's employment patterns have influenced men's participation in domestic activities (Windebank, 2001) and highlights the continuing influences of patriarchal power relations in structuring the experiences of women (Women and Geography Study Group [WGSG], 1997; McKie et al., 2002)—a point not lost on the mothers taking part in my research:

> Yes, I do it. My husband, he has his own business, he's very busy, and he's been spoilt.
> (Charlie and Pete's Mum, Bucks)

There were less clear explanations from fathers as to why they did not juggle the competing demands of employment and participation in family life in a way that many mothers do. Whilst Featherstone (2004) states that many fathers feel trapped in a work culture which prevents participation in family life, none of the fathers spoke of work-related barriers such as a culture of long-hours working (as found in Skinner, 2003) or a lack of family friendly policies which prevented them from taking part in escorting children. Neither did it seem that men simply preferred to be at work rather than escorting children, as some fathers and children expressed disappointment at not participating more in this aspect of family life:

> One of the reasons I would like to get involved (in taking children to school) … as well as
> wanting to walk the dog, is that my daughter loves it (when father takes her). (Daniel's
> Dad, Bucks)

One girl sighed disappointingly:

> Dad, he drives us … sometimes to school, but he's often gone by then. (Kathy, 9, Bucks)

There were aspirations for more involvement of fathers in taking children to and from school and other places, although interestingly the value placed upon this was in relation to benefits to fathers and children, rather than to re-balance a gendered division of labour. McDowell (2003) also discusses how young men valorise involvement in family life and aspire to have a more involved fatherhood than previous generations. However, as this and other research indicates, this aspiration was not always realised in practice (Windebank, 2001). A second, more indirect justification for fathers' lack of involvement relates to broader patterns in everyday parenting and gendered carescapes. Mothers develop local informal social networks with other mothers which are important sources of practical support and information for women (Dyck, 1990; Holloway, 1998). Mothers often co-ordinated car sharing through these networks as one response to the challenge to escort children (Dowling, 2000). However, some fathers stated these social networks justified fathers' non-involvement in organising children's travel:

> My wife makes all the decisions, simply because all the other friends of my daughters have mothers who make decisions. It's easier for them to talk to my wife and vice versa. (Lucy's Dad, Enfield)

This justification for non-involvement is a way of reproducing specific sets of gendered carescapes, which re-inscribe mothers as responsible for children's travel.

However, contemporary societies are characterised by a diversity of family forms and different gendered carescapes and divisions of labour (Bowlby *et al.*, 1997; McDowell, 2004; Mac an Ghaill & Haywood, 2007). In some families fathers played a very significant role, and in one two-parent family and one lone-parent family, fathers had the sole or main responsibility for organising and escorting children. In seven out of 23 families, the division of labour for escorting children was described as equal:

> It's mostly me (who escorts daughter) but if she goes to birthday parties then it's her mother. (Lucy's Dad, Enfield)

> Sometimes ... occasionally I go if he has an eye appointment or a hair dressers appointment, then I go, rather than him going home. I'll say I'll meet him at the school gate, and we'll go from there. But only if there's something happening. Nigel (Dad), he will go if it's his day off, he likes Daddy to come. (Ranj's Mum, Enfield)

These accounts highlight a very different level of participation from fathers than discussed thus far. The day-to-day organisation of escorting was complex and fluid:

> Sometimes, Saturdays if we are both at home, Chris will take him, so I can get on with the housework and the washing. But quite often, Chris is at work on Saturdays, so I will do it. In the week, if there is driving to be done, early evening Chris will have to do it because I am not home from work. So it depends who is home ... it's probably about 50/50. (Ritchie's Mum, Bucks)

This quote illustrates that even within individual families, everyday carescapes and fathers' involvement are fluid, negotiated and change over time and context. As well as escorting their own children to school and other places, two of the four fathers had become volunteers on Safer Routes to School initiatives to reduce congestion at the school gate:

> Graham is the organiser, and Mark is the other driver. The rest is mothers. (Lucy's Dad, Enfield)

> The walking bus, because you (Dad) used to go every Friday. (Ranj's Mum, Enfield)

> Yeah, I used to help out on a Friday morning. (Ranj's Dad, Enfield)

In most of these examples, a prerequisite for fathers' involvement in escorting children was non-standard employment patterns:

> I think the people who can get involved in (the walking bus) are people like us, we both have shift work, so we are often off at that time of day, as opposed to other people rushing off to work. So it was relatively easy for us. (Ranj's Dad, Enfield)

> Our family is different to most people in that we don't work during the day, we get a lot of time off during the week, but not at weekends, or later into the evening. (Vicky's Dad, Enfield)

> Mark (another Dad) walks with me, but he walks on other morning as well. If we have an easy morning, work wise, then we do. We draw pleasure out of walking. It's enjoyable to walk them to school, we benefit from the exercise, and we don't have to spend lots of money in a gym. And for me it works wonders, because I walk the dog, and then I go off for a run in the fields, and then start work. I work from home. (Lucy's Dad, Enfield)

These examples are interesting as they suggest that escorting roles are not taken on by fathers due to a lack of participation in the labour market. This perhaps contests the notion that fathers' increased identification and participation in the domestic sphere is the result of an erosion of a masculine workplace identity and a less secure position within the labour market (Edwards, 2006; Mac an Ghaill & Haywood, 2007). Rather, these fathers had strong—but flexible—links to the labour market (as also found in Brandth & Kvande's 1998 study).

Fun with fathers: escorting children as a masculine concept of care

Different family members discussed how they enjoyed fathers escorting children:

> Plenty of times we have an enjoyable time together ... travelling to school together is just one of the ways to have an enjoyable time with them. (Lucy's Dad, Enfield)

> (I like it as) Dad drives a lot faster than Mum. (Wendy, 7, Bucks)

> Sometimes Mum finds it (driving) hard, because we talk to her on the way there, Dad finds it easier because he's more used to driving. Mum sometimes gets distracted ... Mum can't concentrate as much as Dad can, because he does it so much, he can still talk and drive. (Kathy, 9, Bucks)

Fathers' involvement in the escort of children can create a particular and distinct set of everyday social practices and family experiences and interactions from those children experience with mothers (as also found by Brandth & Kvande, 1998, in relation to looking after small children at home). Cars are not simply functional spaces, but also spaces of sociability for friends and families (Dowling, 2000; Sheller, 2004), and cars were central to some children's accounts of spending time with fathers. Once again, many of the skills or qualities which children associate with fathers' driving are linked to expectations regarding men's behaviours and contemporary masculinities. For example, driving fast, which can be seen as both reflecting defiance and control, is an expression of a particular aspect of contemporary masculinities (Maxwell, 2001; Miller, 2001).

As well as discussing the actual experience of being driven by fathers, children also commented upon features of the different cars that fathers drove:

> Dad's car is a lot higher so it feels different ... better. It makes you feel bigger, and you can see lots more things. (Kathy, 9, Bucks)

> Dad's car, he's got satellite navigation and stuff, so we can type in where to go. (Pete, 9, Bucks)

Some of the accounts here echo the findings of other research, particularly a link between masculinity and technology (Garvey, 2001) and men's preferences for 'side by side' activities, which represent particular masculine forms of intimacy characterised by 'doing something together' (Brandth & Kvande, 1998; Messner, 2001). That fathers do not simply replicate mothers' ways of caring or relating to their children whilst travelling perhaps indicates a distinct, masculine concept of caring for children (Brandth & Kvande, 1998). These men create a more domestic version of masculinity, which although caring, also draws upon everyday practices (such as driving fast, and a reliance upon technology providing the focus for the journey) which are often identified as aspects of hegemonic masculinity (Miller, 2001; Mac an Ghaill & Haywood, 2007). Furthermore, that family members talked mostly positively of fathers' involvement in escorting children indicates that this distinctive masculine value of concept of care is valued by children. In doing so, this may help to legitimate increased involvement of fathers in everyday carescapes.

However, whilst many fathers enjoyed escorting their children to school and other places, their views sometimes reflected those of mothers, in that they often saw themselves as 'taxi services' to escort children:

> I don't mind. When Dad comes (on journey to school), he can carry some of my stuff. (Vicky, 7, Enfield)

> ...We have our uses... (Vicky's Dad, Enfield)

Fathers also discussed some of the problems which they face as men taking part in a role predominantly undertaken by women. Although these fathers were taking on an atypical role and there is often hostility towards non-hegemonic or alternative forms of masculinity (see Connell, 1995; Mac an Ghaill & Haywood, 2007), none of these fathers said they faced criticism or ridicule from their male friends or other fathers for undertaking the escort role. Some fathers described how they had received more of a negative reaction from other mothers than other men. As previously mentioned, local social networks can be highly valuable for mothers. Some fathers taking part in the escort of children stated that they had wanted to participate in these local social networks, but, as men, had often been excluded or found it difficult to make such links. Fathers discussed their experiences of isolation and exclusion outside the school gate:

> In the morning, there are a few (Dads) ... Out of 90 kids in total, there is probably three or four Dads. (Vicky's Dad, Enfield)

> Obviously when I first went there (the school gate), I felt a bit isolated, you do stick out being one of a very small group (of Dad's). (Daniel's Dad, Bucks)

This indicates how despite changes in ideas regarding masculinity and fatherhood, fathers as a social group can still be thought of as existing outside of everyday familial relations or carescapes (Mac an Ghaill & Haywood, 2007). However, some fathers had managed to join these local social networks and discussed the benefits:

> There is a social life amongst the parents (at the school gate), and there are quite a few Dads there. And the school has quite a good extracurricular life as well, with fetes and one another. Anybody who gets involved in doing those things, you get to know one another, that peer group. (Ranj's Dad, Enfield)

> But she's gotten to know other kids in the school, I've gotten to know their parents, and there isn't a problem now. We chat to everyone. But, yes, we are a very small group. (Lucy's Dad, Enfield)

In one family, a mother described one impact of the father undertaking the escort of children—she now found herself more isolated from these local social networks:

> Now I find that, you don't have that contact so much. You say, 'hi', chat to them, maybe arrange to go for a coffee, now you don't do that as much. (Ranj's Mum, Enfield)

In two families, fathers discussed how linking into predominantly female social networks, they have created their own gendered social networks consisting of fathers:

> She's invited to the same parties as her friends, so her friends' Dads can drive her there anyway. They'll drive them there and I will pick them up. (Vicky's Dad, Enfield)

> If they want or need to go out in the evening, once my husband is back, like brownies, we share lifts, and he will always take them there, he alternates with the fathers of the other children who go there. So the wife and I go out and do a class together. (Rachel and Jane's Mum, Bucks)

It is clear that, at least in a limited number of families, fathers undertake the primary role of escorting children and, like mothers, are resourceful in developing their own strategies and networks in response to the challenge to escort children.

Conclusions

Despite growing influences of images of intimacy and involvement of fathers in domestic life, this paper outlines fathers' accounts of their often limited participation in organising and undertaking children's travel. Although women have entered into the labour market, this paper contributes to evidence suggesting this has not necessarily led to an equally profound shift in the participation of fathers in the domestic sphere. Similarly, despite broader changes in the role of fathers and expectations surrounding masculinity, which are witnessed in other aspects of men's lives (see Mac an Ghaill & Haywood, 2007), this paper adds to the evidence which suggests this has had limited influence in everyday gendered social practices and carescapes in relation to escorting children. Indeed whilst the findings here do not reflect what Crompton et al. (2005) describe a 'glacial' pace of change, they do perhaps resonate more with

Pilcher's notion of a 'resilience of inequalities' (2000, p. 774) in relation to gendered carescapes.

The findings also contribute to evidence mapping the diversity of contemporary UK fatherhood experiences (McDowell, 2003; Edwards, 2006). The accounts here suggest very diverse roles for fathers and different expectations about participation in children's lives. Whilst some fathers have very limited engagement, in a limited number of cases, fathers have the primary responsibility for organising and undertaking the escort of children. Some feel isolated in their role as escort, whilst others have linked with and developed social networks to help carry out escorting. The different and diverse everyday social practices which constitute fatherhood in some families reflect a more informal, negotiated and mediated position of fatherhood in contemporary societies. The changing economic contexts have enabled some fathers to take a greater role in escorting children.

Contributing to debates about gendered divisions of labour, the paper demonstrates how carescapes are not only gendered in terms of the amount of caring undertaken but also the type of caring offered. These accounts show escorting children as a role within fatherhood is different and distinct to the ways in which it is undertaken by mothers. Escorting children does not necessarily mean a break with hegemonic forms of masculinity, nor do these fathers appear to be criticised by other men for their involvement in escorting children. Rather, fathers' involvement in the escort of children creates distinct everyday experiences from those with mothers, creating a masculine form of caring (as also explored by Brandth & Kvande, 1998). Importantly, fathers and children place high value on fathers' participation, suggesting this form of caring may be positive for children and families. Interestingly, the value attached to fathers' participation focuses on benefits to fathers and children—as a distinct masculine form of caring—rather than a desire or strategy to develop more gender-equal carescapes.

References

Barker, J. (2003) Passengers or political actors? Children's participation in transport policy and the micro political geographies of the family, *Space and Polity*, 7(2), 135–152.

Barker, J. & Weller, S. (2003) 'Is it fun?' Developing children centred research methods, *International Journal of Sociology and Social Policy*, 23(1), 33–58.

Beckmann, J. (2001) Automobility—a social problem and theoretical concept, *Environment and Planning D: Society and Space*, 19, 593–607.

Bowlby, S., Gregory, S. & McKie, L. (1997) 'Doing home': patriarchy, caring and space, *Women's Studies International Forum*, 20(3), 343–350.

Brandth, B. & Kvande, E. (1998) Masculinity and childcare: the reconstruction of fathering, *Sociological Review*, 46(2), 293–313.

Butera, K. (2006) Manhunt: the challenge of enticing men to participate in a study on friendship, *Qualitative Enquiry*, 12, 1262–1282.

Castelain-Meunier, C. (2002) The place of fatherhood and the parental role: tensions, ambivalence and contradictions, *Current Sociology*, 50, 185–201.

Connell, R. (1995) *Masculinities* (Cambridge, Polity).

Crompton, R., Borckmann, B. & Lyonette, C. (2005) Attitudes, women's employment and the domestic division of labour: a cross-national analysis in two waves, *Work, Employment and Society*, 19, 213–223.

DfT (2004) *Transport statistics bulletin: National Travel Survey 2003 final results* (London, The Stationery Office).

DfT (2005) *Focus on personal travel* (London, The Stationery Office).

DfT (2007) *Transport trends: 2007 edition.* Available online at: http://www.dft.gov.uk/pgr/statistics/datatablepublications/trends/current/ (accessed 14 December 2007).

Dowling, R. (2000) Cultures of mothering and car use in suburban Sydney: a preliminary investigation, *Geoforum*, 31, 345–353.

Dyck, I. (1990) Space, time and renegotiating motherhood: an exploration of the domestic workplace, *Environment and Planning D: Society and Space*, 8, 459–483.

Edwards, T. (2006) *Cultures of masculinity* (London, Routledge).

Featherstone, B. (2004) Fathers matter: a research review, *Children and Society*, 18, 312–319.

Garvey, P. (2001) Driving, drinking and daring in Norway, in: D. Miller (Ed.) *Car cultures* (Oxford, Berg), 133–152.

Hillman, M., Adams, J. & Whitelegg, J. (1990) *One false move: a study of children's independent mobility* (London, Policy Studies Institute).

Holloway, S. (1998) Local childcare cultures: moral geographies of mothering and the social organisation of preschool education, *Gender, Place and Culture*, 5(1), 29–53.

Jones, P. & Bradshaw, R. (2000) *The family and the school run: what would make a real difference?* (Basingstoke, AA Foundation for Road Safety Research).

Joshi, M., MacLean, M. & Carter, W. (1999) Children's journey to school: spatial skills, knowledge and perceptions of the environment, *British Journal of Developmental Psychology*, 17, 125–139.

Laurie, N., Dwyer, C., Holloway, S. & Smith, F. (1999) *Geographies of new femininities* (Harlow, Longman).

Law, R. (1999) Beyond 'women and transport': towards new geographies of gender and daily mobility, *Progress in Human Geography*, 23(4), 567–588.

Mac an Ghaill, M. & Haywood, C. (2007) *Gender, culture and society: contemporary femininities and masculinities* (Basingstoke, Macmillan Palgrave).

Maxwell, S. (2001) Negotiations of car use in everyday life, in: D. Miller (Ed.) *Car cultures* (Oxford, Berg), 203–222.

Mayall, B. (1994) Children in action at home and at school, in: B. Mayall (Ed.) *Children's childhoods: observed and experienced* (London, Falmer), 114–127.

McAllister, R. & Grey, C. (2006) Low vision: mobility and independence training for the early years child, *Early Years Development and Care*, 177(8), 839–852.

McDowell, L. (2003) *Redundant masculinities: employment change and white working class youth* (Oxford, Blackwell).

McDowell, L. (2004) Work, workfare, work/life balance and an ethic of care, *Progress in Human Geography*, 28(2), 145–163.

McKie, L., Gregory, S. & Bowlby, S. (2002) Shadow times: the temporal and spatial frameworks and experiences of caring and working, *Sociology*, 36(4), 897–924.

Meaton, J. & Kingham, M. (1998) Children's perceptions of transport modes: car culture in the classroom, *World Transport Policy and Practice*, 4(2), 12–16.

Messner, M. (2001) Friendship, intimacy and sexuality, in: S. Whitehead & F. Barrett (Eds) *The masculinities reader* (Cambridge, Polity), 253–265.

Miller, D. (2001) Driven societies, in: D. Miller (Ed.) *Car cultures* (Oxford, Berg), 1–33.

O'Brien, M., Jones, D. & Sloan, D. (2000) Children's independent spatial mobility in the urban public realm, *Childhood*, 7(3), 257–277.

Pilcher, J. (2000) Domestic divisions of labour in the twentieth century: 'change slow-a-coming', *Work, Employment and Society*, 14, 771–780.

RCEP (1994) *Transport and the environment* (London, HMSO).

Rye, T. (2002) Travel plans: do they work? *Transport Policy*, 9, 287–298.

Saracho, O. (2007) Fathers and young children's literacy experiences in a family environment, *Early Years Development and Care,* 177(4), 403–415.

Sheller, M. (2004) Mobile publics: beyond the network perspective, *Environment and Planning D: Society and Space,* 22(1), 39–52.

Skinner, C. (2003) *How parents co-ordinate childcare, education and work.* JRF findings ref no. 593 (York, Joseph Rowntree Foundation).

Turner, J. & Grieco, M. (1998) Gender and time poverty: the neglected social policy implications of gendered time, transport and travel, paper presented at the *International Conference on Time Use,* Institute of Luneberg, Germany, 6 April.

Urry, J. (2000) *Sociology beyond societies: mobilities for the 21st century* (London, Routledge).

Valentine, G. & McKendrick, J. (1997) Children's outdoor play: exploring parental concerns about children's safety and the changing nature of childhood, *Geoforum,* 28(2), 219–235.

West, A., Noden, P., Edge, A. & David, M. (1998) Parental involvement in education in and out of school, *British Educational Research Journal,* 24(4), 461–484.

WGSG (1997) *Feminist geographies: explorations in diversity and difference* (Harlow, Longman).

Windebank, J. (2001) Dual-earner couples in Britain and France: gender divisions of domestic labour and parenting work in different welfare states, *Work, Employment and Society,* 15(2), 269–290.

Index